Lewandowski has created an easy-to-use manual people can use to help manage p.... by following the simple exercises included, they may better understand the perpetuating factors contributing to their pain so they may embrace effective strategies for managing fatigue, thoughts, behaviors, and suffering. The book's information about working with doctors will prove invaluable, and by using the recommendations included, people with pain will be able to get more out of every medical visit. This book will help those with chronic pain ultimately live more satisfying and productive lives.

—B. Eliot Cole, MD, MPA, executive director of the American Society of Pain Educators

This is the best self help book on chronic pain that I have seen. It is clearly written, has many helpful suggestions, and is evidenced based. This is an outstanding source of helpful information written by an astute clinician and one of the nation's leaders in chronic pain management.

—William O'Donohue, Ph.D., Nicholas Cummings Professor of Organized Behavioral Healthcare Delivery in the Department of Psychology at the University of Nevada, Reno

Pain is the ubiquitous and often debilitating accompaniment to most chronic illnesses. Lewandowski has written an important, clinically sound, and remarkably user-friendly self-treatment approach that can be of much needed benefit to pain sufferers. It is strongly recommended.

—Nicholas A. Cummings, Ph.D., Sc.D., past president of the American Psychological Association; distinguished professor emeritus of clinical psychology at the University of Nevada, Reno; and president, of the Cummings Foundation for Behavioral Health

The Behavioral Assessment of Pain questionnaire has been a great asset to our practice. Patients appreciate its comprehensiveness and the information gathered makes a significant impact on the interdisciplinary treatment plan. It is a very efficient way to gain an understanding of how chronic pain has impacted the patient's lives and helps to individualize care.

—Robert P. Trombley, Ph.D., director of pain psychology at the Advanced Pain Centers of Alaska

I have been using the BAP for four years to help neurosurgeons screen prospective back pain patients for morphine pumps and nerve stimulators. The BAP identifies outcome indicators which are meaningful for both surgeons and patients. I cannot imagine attempting a valid pain evaluation without the BAP.

—Richard Whitten, Ph.D., Great Plains Psychological Services in Souix Falls, SD

I have found the Behavioral Assessment of Pain questionnaire (BAP) to have high face validity with my patients. It is a terrific test. The test results are very useful and it is easy to administer.

—Avrum Green, Ph.D., psychologist in Owensound, ON, Canada

The Chronic Pain Care Workbook *is clearly written, with many self-exams and few statistics. It covers all aspects of chronic pain, and it will serve as a useful tool to help the reader regain normal function and minimize the impact of pain on daily life. The book can also serve as an adjunct to a more structured pain management program…a useful addition to the self-help literature on chronic pain management.*

—Book review by John D. Loeser, MD, professor of neurological surgery and anesthesiology at the University of Washington

The
Chronic Pain Care
WORKBOOK

A Self-Treatment Approach
to Pain Relief Using the
Behavioral Assessment of
Pain Questionnaire

MICHAEL J. LEWANDOWSKI, PH.D.

New Harbinger Publications, Inc.

Publisher's Note

This publication is designed to provide accurate and authoritative information in regard to the subject matter covered. It is sold with the understanding that the publisher is not engaged in rendering psychological, financial, legal, or other professional services. If expert assistance or counseling is needed, the services of a competent professional should be sought.

Care has been taken to confirm the accuracy of the information presented and to describe generally accepted practices. However, the authors, editors, and publisher are not responsible for errors or omissions or for any consequences from application of the information in this book and make no warranty, express or implied, with respect to the contents of the publication.

The authors, editors, and publisher have exerted every effort to ensure that any drug selection and dosage set forth in this text are in accordance with current recommendations and practice at the time of publication. However, in view of ongoing research, changes in government regulations, and the constant flow of information relating to drug therapy and drug reactions, the reader is urged to check the package insert for each drug for any change in indications and dosage and for added warnings and precautions. This is particularly important when the recommended agent is a new or infrequently employed drug.

Some drugs and medical devices presented in this publication may have Food and Drug Administration (FDA) clearance for limited use in restricted research settings. It is the responsibility of the health care provider to ascertain the FDA status of each drug or device planned for use in their clinical practice.

Thought evaluation form on page 108 from Judith S. Beck, Ph.D., "Worksheet Packet," Bala Cynwyd, PA, Beck Institute for Cognitive therapy and Research, Copyright © 1996 (Revised 2006). Adapted with permission.

Opioid Risk Tool on page 95 from Lynn Webster, MD, © 2005. Reprinted with permission.

Distributed in Canada by Raincoast Books

Copyright © 2006 by Michael Lewandowski
New Harbinger Publications, Inc.
5674 Shattuck Avenue
Oakland, CA 94609
www.newharbinger.com

Cover design by Amy Shoup; Acquired by Tesilya Hanauer;
Text design by Tracy Marie Carlson; Edited by Jessica Beebe

All Rights Reserved. Printed in the United States of America.

Library of Congress Cataloging-in-Publication Data

Lewandowski, Michael J.
   The chronic pain care workbook : a self-treatment approach to pain relief using the behavioral assessment of pain questionnaire / Michael J. Lewandowski.
      p. cm.
   ISBN-13: 978-1-57224-470-2
   ISBN-10: 1-57224-470-4
   1. Chronic pain—Treatment. 2. Chronic pain—Alternative treatment. 3. Self-care, Health. I. Title.
RB127.L49 2006
616'.0472—dc22
                      2006024503

15 14 13

10   9   8   7   6

This book is dedicated to my wife, Kristin. No words can adequately express my appreciation for her love, support, and incredible wisdom.

Contents

PART I
WHAT IS CHRONIC PAIN?

PART 2
BEHAVIORAL ASSESSMENT OF PAIN

Foreword

The Chronic Pain Care Workbook holds within its pages a unique step-by-step approach to help people who are suffering from chronic pain. Dr. Lewandowski teaches effective pain management with simplicity and guides the reader with self-assessment quizzes that lead to individualized pain self-management recommendations.

The field of pain management has been calling for efforts to tailor treatment to fit the needs of different kinds of people suffering from chronic pain. This book answers that call. Through a series of quizzes, readers build a Pain Scorecard that shows what factors maintain or worsen their pain experience. The Pain Scorecard allows readers to focus their treatment efforts where they will be most effective.

I have worked for decades to counteract the prevailing medical view of a person as a body with a set of symptoms. A person is not simply a diagnosis. A person—a real person—is the product of mind, body, and spirit. Biological, psychological, and social factors all come together in the individual. That meeting is keenly and expertly addressed in *The Chronic Pain Care Workbook*. This workbook offers exactly what people in pain need: a comprehensive biopsychosocial perspective.

In my work at the UCLA Pain Management Center, I saw people in every type of pain imaginable—from A to Z, from arthritis to zygapophyseal joint pain. Each person's experience of pain was unique. Yet the treatment was usually a series of interventional, isolated polytherapies that had little relation to each other, let alone to the patient.

Too often, people in pain are stuck in limbo. With no diagnosis, there is no prognosis. They feel that without knowing what is wrong, there is no way to make it right. They are waiting for a doctor to take control. But, in reality, they need to take that control for themselves. This book not only shows people how to take back control, it also empowers them to do so.

In a day and age when science is making huge leaps in the molecular, biological, and pharmacological aspects of pain, we are woefully stagnant when it comes to understanding the unique person who is experiencing pain. The totality of the human condition is remarkably complex. Yet we keep trying to simplify it, reducing it to the physical, to the detriment of those truly suffering.

So maybe the key to progress in pain management lies not with science but with people. Individuals with pain can be empowered to assess themselves from a biopsychosocial perspective and adopt a self-management approach. *The Chronic Pain Care Workbook* guides readers down their unique paths of self-management.

—Richard Kroening, MD, Ph.D.

Author's Note

Dr. Richard Kroening passed away prior to the publication of this book. The foreword to this book contains his last observations about people suffering from chronic pain. I was extremely fortunate to have him as my mentor. He changed my life and will be missed.

Preface

Too many people suffer from chronic pain. They aren't *living* with chronic pain; they are *suffering*, truly suffering. I know because I work with people in pain every day in my practice as a behavioral psychologist. Every day, I see people who have given up hope, given up control, given up living. I see them bowed under the weight of pain, so bent they no longer bother to look up and see the world around them. I see them worn like sandstone scoured by the constant onslaught of weather, too ravaged to see their own beauty. They are referred to me because their medications aren't cutting it or because their doctors haven't been able to help them. But they usually don't expect much improvement, not really. They feel they've tried everything already, and they're tired. They're angry, confused, and numb. But they all want to feel better.

And the good news? They can. *You* can. Every person dealing with chronic pain can feel better. They—and you—can regain control by actively participating in the management of chronic pain. It is time to decrease the control pain has on your quality of life by taking that control back. You may have chronic pain, but chronic pain doesn't have to have you.

This book is intended for people suffering from persistent and chronic pain who want to regain control of the quality of their lives and feel better.

The causes of chronic pain are many. This book attempts to not only look at the physical and biological causes of pain but also examine the emotional, psychological, and social consequences of having chronic pain. Researchers in the field of pain management call this approach the *biopsychosocial* view of pain, and it is this approach and model that I use in *The Chronic Pain Care Workbook.*

While the biopsychosocial model is the epitome of our understanding of chronic pain, it is not a magic bullet. There are no simple solutions. I'm sorry to say that this book doesn't have all the answers. You won't feel better just by holding it in your hands or sticking it under your pillow. You'll need to read it and decide for yourself what ideas, methods, and strategies can work for you.

Following the recommendations in this workbook and applying its lessons to your life, however, will make you feel better. The proof is in the doing. In my pain management practice, I have worked with more than five thousand people who have chronic pain. They have taught me much about the human capacity for growth and change. They have also shown me that chronic pain is a uniquely personal experience. No two people experience chronic pain the same way, even if their pain is caused by the same type of injury.

Doing the work in this workbook means being an active participant rather than a passive recipient of treatment and taking charge of your quality of life and ability to function. Too many people with chronic pain give up participating in their own physical well-being, deferring to those they consider more knowledgeable. Since most authorities on chronic pain view pain as a biopsychosocial experience, it's unrealistic to expect one domain (medicine) to fix it. Yet many people in pain continue to search for the cure—working exclusively from the biological perspective—only to feel frustrated, angry, depressed, anxious, and isolated.

Pain support groups are growing throughout the country as people seek support and search for meaning in their experiences of pain. The primary tenet of many of these groups is that you may not have a choice as to whether you have chronic pain, but you do have a choice in how you react to pain. *The Chronic Pain Care Workbook* will present you with more options for coping with pain. This book will teach you a set of tools and coping skills you can use to improve your psychological and social as well as physical well-being.

If you want to improve, really improve, you must act. I can't stress this enough. Action is absolutely necessary for improvement. Not intentions, not knowledge, not hope, but real action and the effort that goes with it. Reading this book is the ideal first step.

THIS BOOK IS NOT A MEDICAL REVIEW OF YOUR CONDITION

The self-management approach to chronic pain is all about knowing yourself. The more you know about why you hurt, the more you can learn about how you hurt, and the better you can understand how you can hurt less. This book will help you explore the physical causes of your pain, assess your current perception of your medical care, and offer you some ideas and strategies for getting more information if you need it.

However, keep in mind that nothing in this book is meant to be a medical review of your condition. If you experience any of the following conditions, consult a physician as soon as possible.

- Loss of bowel or bladder control

- Loss of sexual function or numbness in the groin

- Weakness in the legs and feet

- Throbbing and aching pain that wakes you from sleep

- Serious physical trauma

- Excruciating pain with new symptoms and new locations

- Problems with medications or increased use of alcohol for pain relief

Acknowledgments

So much of what I have learned over the past twenty-three years in the field of pain management has come from listening to the thousands of people who have shared their unique experience of pain and suffering. While I cannot mention them all, a special thanks to Kristian Darling, Bruce Furneaux, Lisa Schreiner, and Linda Springfield.

For their wisdom and guidance, I also wish to thank University of Nevada professors Dr. James Mikawa, Dr. Bob Peterson, Dr. Duane Varble, Dr. Lyle Warner, Dr. D. Koh, Dr. David Antonuccio, Dr. William O'Donahue, and Dr. Paul McReynolds. The statistical assistance of Dr. William Meredith at the University of California, Berkeley, was critical in the development of the Behavioral Assessment of Pain questionnaire. Without the help of each of these people, none of this would have been possible.

A special thanks to Dr. Blake Tearnan, friend and colleague, who was instrumental in the development and birth of the Behavioral Assessment of Pain questionnaire.

I thank Cindie Geddes at Flying Hand, who was invaluable with editing and whose emotional support during this process I greatly appreciated. Advice and feedback from my friends Michael Johnson and Sandy Beckett kept me on track, and I thank them.

Thank you also to Tesilya Hanauer, acquistions editor at New Harbinger Publications, who believed in the project and gave it life. Many thanks to my agent, Nancy Crossman, who worked so effectively with the staff at New Harbinger to make this a reality.

Finally, I thank my mother and father, Theresa and Leonard Lewandowski, who encouraged me to continue my education and perhaps someday write a book.

Introduction

My passion for helping people take control of their pain has led me in a variety of directions—all with the common destination of helping those in pain. I am a licensed clinical psychologist and president of Pain Assessment Resources, a company that assists health care professionals who work with people who have chronic pain. I have extensive training—and, more importantly, a great deal of experience—in the application of psychological principles to problems in medicine.

Early in my professional career, I was extremely fortunate to be trained and mentored by Dr. Richard Kroening, former director of the Pain Management Program at the University of California, Los Angeles. He was the first to show me the therapeutic value of a team approach in working with people suffering from chronic pain and the first to introduce the importance of understanding pain as a *biopsychosocial* experience.

Since completing my Ph.D. in 1990 at the University of Nevada, I have worked exclusively with people suffering from chronic medical and pain conditions. While I was director of the Behavioral Medicine Department for a pain management program in Nevada, the program achieved the highest level of accreditation from the Commission on Accreditation of Rehabilitation Facilities. In addition to my clinical, administrative, and legal experience working with chronic pain sufferers, I have conducted, presented, and published original scientific research in the area of chronic pain at conferences throughout the world.

All of my experience has been poured into the development of a pain assessment tool, the Behavioral Assessment of Pain (BAP) questionnaire, which is used in pain management programs worldwide. The BAP has become the cornerstone of my clinical work, and it will help guide you along your pain management journey.

WHY I WROTE THIS BOOK

One of the greatest needs in the field of chronic pain management is teaching people how to manage their pain using a self-directed, self-help approach. *The Chronic Pain Care Workbook* offers just that, allowing you to answer specific questions about your unique pain experience. These questions address everything from counterproductive ideas and beliefs about pain to depression, anger, and anxiety; from sleep disturbance to activity avoidance. Answering all these questions will lead you to a personalized pain management profile that outlines your personal strengths in coping with pain and gives you specific treatment recommendations.

The Chronic Pain Care Workbook provides a simple program for you to regain control of your life by taking control of your pain. But unlike too many self-help books on pain management, this book is not about quick fixes, fads, or platitudes. This workbook was developed from my two decades of experience in pain management, and the recommended treatments are based on the latest clinical research in the field of pain management. The book incorporates real-world data and scientific expertise to offer you a powerful new lease on life.

Before we get started, take a moment to think about your goals. How do you want to be different? What do you want to change? Here is a list of goals I had in mind when I wrote the book. Let's see if we are a good match.

The Chronic Pain Care Workbook will help you:

- Learn more about what influences your pain

- Improve the quality of your life

- Get back in the driver's seat of life, not the backseat

- Sleep better and wake feeling more refreshed and alive

- Improve your relationships with family, friends, and coworkers

- Be in a better mood

- Return to productive work and meaningful play

- Get real about the negative impact of your pain

- Understand the relationship between stress, psychological factors, and physical symptoms

- Increase your ability to exercise

- Increase your physical activity

- Increase your ability to care for yourself

- Develop basic relaxation skills to improve pain management

- Reduce how often you complain about pain

- Learn thinking skills to deal with pain

- Learn to divert your attention away from pain

- Decrease the amount of pity and attention you get from family and friends

- Improve sexual functioning

- Find ways to meet your emotional needs

- Learn to be more assertive

- Feel less helpless

- Learn to recognize improvements and accomplishments

- Recognize the impact that your behavior has on others

- Become more active and less dependent on others

In the end, the number one reason I wrote this book is to encourage positive change. While I can't simulate one-on-one care, I hope to make this a personal journey toward a better and more active life. A self-management strategy that monitors improvement (through exercises, graphs, and writing) is the most efficient and beneficial program I have found, one that lends itself quite well to the workbook format.

HOW TO USE THIS BOOK

Not all chronic pain is curable, but all chronic pain is manageable. *The Chronic Pain Care Workbook* will help you decrease the effect of pain on your day-to-day life. Throughout this book, I will act as your partner and validating collaborator. But I'm not the expert here. You are the expert. Nobody knows your pain like you do. I'll share what I have learned from my education and training and from people who suffer from chronic pain. If I can help you look at your pain differently, develop some new tools, and perhaps sharpen some existing ones, I will have accomplished my goal. But only you can choose what to build with those tools.

Working through this book is a journey of discovery. This book seeks to help you find out which factors do and do not work in the management of *your* pain. In the end, you will have a unique self-management plan unlike anyone else's.

Vince Lombardi, Hall of Fame football coach for the Green Bay Packers, once said that the only place you find success before work is in the dictionary. Pain management takes work, so you need to be up for the challenge. Self-management is an active process, so you can't sit on the sidelines if you want to feel better. No one else is going to take charge of managing your pain, because no one else is experiencing what you are experiencing. But while you may be alone in your experience of your pain, you are not alone in your quest for a better quality of life. We will work together through this workbook to help you take charge of your experience, your pain, your life.

The self-management approach is powerful for two simple reasons:

1. You are the expert. You know the nuances and evolution of your pain. You can tell subtle changes, for better or worse.

2. Participating actively in changing your pain experience helps you attribute success to your own competence and not to external authority. It makes you more motivated. Rather than relying on outside forces to improve your lot, you can take charge and know you are capable of managing your own experience.

While this book will explore a variety of factors that can increase your pain (such as physical tissue damage, inactivity, thoughts, poor sleep, mood problems, the way you do things, the reactions of others, and your responses to pain), no one thing is likely to be causing all of your pain problems. Understanding your pain is like doing a jigsaw puzzle. First you look at all the pieces to make sure you're not missing any. Then you start experimenting with how the pieces fit together. Finally, you can see the big picture. You may not have all the pieces today, since modern medicine can bring wonderful advances, but by starting the process you can begin to see what emerges.

The big picture of pain management is made up of information and skills you can find in this book. With these tools, you can build a new, better life.

HOW THIS BOOK IS ORGANIZED

You'll begin your journey of taking control of your pain by learning to understand your pain, including where it comes from and how you react. In part 1, I cover the basics of pain.

Part 2 takes a close look at how you have dealt with chronic pain and its impact on your life. You'll assess how the biological, psychological, and social domains influence your pain, and you'll learn tools for better managing your pain experience. Your response to the questions will reveal your personal strengths for coping with pain and also those areas that may need more attention.

While there are a variety of programs to help you manage your pain, changing how you behave and changing how you think are at the heart of the most effective. Research shows that the most effective pain management approaches share the following characteristics:

- Increasing your physical activity through graduated movement and exercise

- Altering the ways you do things, while avoiding extremes

- Learning fatigue management techniques (including good sleep habits)

- Challenging unproductive thoughts and ideas about pain

- Learning assertiveness skills

- Learning relaxation skills

All of these skills will be discussed or taught in this book.

Part 3 focuses on handling setbacks and maintaining your treatment gains.

Part 4 includes your Pain Scorecard. As you complete the exercises in each chapter, you will transfer your results to the Pain Scorecard so that you can see the big picture. The Pain Scorecard can tell you what specific areas you need to work on and what areas you are handling well. You can then focus on the areas of concern and spend your energy where it will do the most good.

The Pain Scorecard is also set up to show any changes you have made. By answering the questions once more after you have started to make changes in your life, you will be able to see your progress. The differences between your "before" and "after" scores will show you the distance you have come.

The Pain Scorecard can also be a helpful document to share with physicians, psychologists, physical therapists, family members—anyone who is part of your pain management team. This way you can all start from the same place, and all work toward the same goal, with full knowledge of your particular pain management strengths and struggles.

Resources for pain management—such as how to find a therapist or physician, obtain answers to medical questions, and locate support groups—are included at the end of the book.

SELF-MONITORING IS A KEY TO PAIN RELIEF AND MANAGEMENT

As you work through this book, I hope that you will see real-life evidence that the self-management approach is improving your quality of life. This evidence will make it easier for you to continue. Managing pain can be hard work, and you are more likely to persevere if you remind yourself why you are learning and practicing new skills. Keep your goals (which you'll list in chapter 4) handy—put a copy in your wallet, use it as a bookmark, tack it up on the fridge. While you don't need to dwell on the negatives of chronic pain, do keep in mind that your pain interferes with a variety of factors in your life: sleep, participation in valued activities, mood. Reviewing these negative effects—along with the benefits of self-management—helps you stay motivated.

Adding consequences to your goals will only strengthen your resolve. In many ways, we humans are simple creatures. We respond well to rewards. As you go through your self-management program, remember to build rewards into your system. For example, allow yourself to relax after exercise, treat yourself to a nice warm bath at the end of a hard day, and pat yourself on the back when you accomplish even the smallest of gains. This will help you maintain your self-management practice.

CREATING YOUR UNIQUE PAIN PROFILE

If chronic pain is like a puzzle, it often feels as if many of the pieces are missing. We are going to start by finding some of the pieces and getting them in place, just as you might group all the straight-edged pieces in a jigsaw puzzle before putting them together. Throughout this book, you will answer questions that will help define pieces of that puzzle. These very same questions have been asked of more than a thousand other people suffering from chronic pain. Their answers have given a normal or typical range for responses, and they serve as a baseline by which to judge your experience.

Chronic pain, however, is not a constant, consistent experience. Fluctuations, variations, and deviations are all part of the picture. Your pain may be worse on some days and better on others. At various times (of the day, night, or week), you may answer questions differently, and that is okay. When you respond to the questions with your average or typical experience, you will get the most accurate pieces to your particular puzzle.

Your responses to the questions will help you measure your progress as you continue with this program. Yes, it will take time—just as it takes time to create a productive garden or a fine wine—but it will be time well spent. These questions were developed through years of study and analysis in order to help you discover your unique pain profile and help you find your optimal approach to taking control of your pain and thereby your life.

GETTING FURTHER HELP

While you can use the advice and strategies offered in this book on your own, *The Chronic Pain Care Workbook* does not ignore the benefits offered by medical and psychological professionals. To find professionals in your area with expertise in pain management, go to my Web site (www.PainCareWorkbook. com) or see Resources at the end of this book.

PART I

WHAT IS CHRONIC PAIN?

Chances are, if you have picked up this book, you are familiar with pain. You have probably been struggling with pain for months or even years. Normally, pain is temporary. We can be thankful for that. But if you have been experiencing pain for more than three months, you have chronic pain.

The common denominator for people who experience chronic pain is suffering. Your quality of life and ability to function has likely been dramatically affected by your pain. You have probably seen a number of doctors and therapists who have tried their best to solve your pain problem. They have likely administered numerous medications, tests, and procedures, but your suffering continues. You may even feel that the medical system has failed you.

I want to present to you what I have learned over the past twenty-three years of working in the field of pain management as a behavioral psychologist. I hope that after reading *The Chronic Pain Care Workbook*, you will be armed with new ideas, information, and strategies to reduce your suffering and return to a higher level of physical functioning. I hope you feel better.

CHAPTER 1

Chronic Pain Care Basics

Put simply, chronic pain is any pain that lasts more than three months. If you are suffering from chronic pain, you are not alone. A variety of studies have looked at the effects of pain on individuals and society. Key among these is a 1999 study by Elliott and colleagues. Some of their findings include:

- Over 50 million people in the United States suffer from chronic pain, yet most medical students don't take a single course focused on treating pain.

- At least 45 percent of Americans will seek care or treatment for persistent pain at some point in their lives.

- A recent poll showed three out of four people surveyed either suffered from pain themselves or had a close family member or friend who was suffering.

- Pain is the most common reason Americans seek medical care and is a leading cause of disability in the United States.

- Chronic pain takes a greater toll on the United States economy in health insurance claims than any other chronic condition, including heart disease, hypertension, and diabetes.

- Pain is the leading cause of lost productivity and costs employers over $80 billion a year.

- As the baby boomers continue to age, the problem will only get worse.

There is a huge variety of chronic pain problems. The most common types of chronic pain I see in my practice are low back pain, fibromyalgia, myofascial pain, complex regional pain syndrome, neuropathic pain, chronic headaches (including tension, migraine, and cluster headaches), arthritis, and temporomandibular disorders.

If you have persistent pain, you undoubtedly want to feel better. You want to break free from the hold that pain has on your life. Breaking free from the control pain wields over you is even more important than breaking free of the pain itself. You can live with pain, but only if you can modify its impact upon your life. This book is all about regaining your life. If you realize that you have reached an impasse in effectively coping with pain, and you want to find better ways to manage it, this book is written especially for you.

ACUTE AND CHRONIC PAIN

A key element in pain management is the distinction between acute and chronic pain. *Acute pain* lasts from the moment of injury to about twelve weeks. *Chronic pain* lasts longer than twelve weeks. Acute pain can be mild to severe, similar to chronic pain, but acute pain conditions are easily diagnosable, meaning the source of the pain can be discovered. This is not typically the case with chronic pain. Each type of pain needs to be treated differently. Problems occur when health care providers treat chronic pain as if it were an acute pain problem. In fact, mistreatment can inadvertently perpetuate the pain.

Acute pain can be useful as a warning signal. It is an alarm system that alerts the body to respond quickly to threats. People who are born with *congenital analgesia*, a condition in which they feel no pain, actually suffer shorter life spans. They can't feel when they have broken bones or acquired infections. They don't have the warning systems that alert most people to seek medical help.

Resting and protecting a painful area following an acute injury is *adaptive*; it eventually increases your ability to live your life, in this case by allowing your body to heal. However, reliance on rest in the case of chronic pain is often *maladaptive*; it eventually decreases your ability to live your life. Acute pain goes away, so the rest period has an end in sight. When the pain doesn't go away, you need to find a way to live with it. So do the people around you. The social component of chronic pain can be huge.

CAUSES AND EFFECTS OF CHRONIC PAIN

When you consider the causes of chronic pain, you probably think about the beginning, an injury, trauma, or accident—the biological factors. And biological factors are definitely important. Some types of pain are *neuropathic*, that is, caused by injury or damage to nerve tissue or by malfunctioning nerve signals. This is typically felt as burning, shooting, and stabbing pain; examples include sciatica or a pinched nerve. Other types of pain are *nociceptive*, or caused by inflammation, disease, or injury to certain tissues such as muscles, tendons, or ligaments. Knowing the difference is important because each type of pain can react to different treatments. But it's also important to examine the emotional, social, and psychological aftershocks of chronic pain—the impact on not only the person in pain, but also the people around that person. Family, friends, and coworkers may all be affected by your chronic pain.

Research has shown that pain can be modified to reduce the associated misery. This is the good news. You have the power to make significant changes in your experience of chronic pain. In this book, you will look beyond the physical problems that have led up to your life with chronic pain; you will consider all the parts of your life that have been affected by your chronic pain. We are going to examine those factors that are contributing to, maintaining, and exacerbating your pain experience. We will also look at different strategies to put you back in the driver's seat of your life. For the millions of people suffering from chronic pain, a new focus on self-management of pain is long overdue.

EXERCISE 1.1: DO YOU HAVE CHRONIC PAIN?

Answer the following questions to see if your pain is truly chronic.

Have you had pain for more than three months?   (yes) no

Has your pain interfered with your daily life?   (yes) no

Is your quality of life unacceptable to you due to your pain?   (yes) no

Are you unable to be active and function at an acceptable level due to your pain? (yes) no

If you answered yes to these questions, chronic pain is a real problem in your life, and this book can help.

PAIN MYTHS AND FALLACIES

The myths involved with chronic pain could fill a book all on their own. Partners for Understanding Pain, a consortium of more than fifty organizations that have an interest in pain and its effects, commissioned a telephone survey of 1,000 American adults which revealed that many held beliefs contrary to established facts about pain and pain management (American Chronic Pain Association 2002). Although pain is the primary cause of disability in the United States, almost two-thirds of those surveyed thought disability claims were caused by other medical conditions, not pain. Even though most physicians have very little training in pain management, the vast majority of people surveyed believed strongly that their primary care physician could effectively diagnose and treat any pain problem they encountered. Although 80 percent of people who have chronic pain are between twenty-four and sixty-four, most of those surveyed thought the typical chronic pain patient was sixty-five or older. And even though most pain medications rarely cause addiction, over three-quarters of the respondents expressed concern about addiction from prescribed pain medications.

Every day I hear people's ideas and beliefs about living with pain. Some people tell me at the beginning of my interview that they don't know why they are seeing a psychologist for their pain. They have real pain, and they just need to find the right doctor or combination of treatments. But there are a few common ideas and beliefs about pain that are simply wrong. Here are my top four.

Rest is best.   Rest *is* best—but for acute pain, not chronic pain. With acute pain, such as pain caused by a pulled muscle, rest is what allows the injury to heal. But rest is definitely not best for chronic pain.

Rest is best is a belief people build from their real experiences dealing with acute injuries and pain. But if your pain is going to be with you for years, maybe the rest of your life, are you really prepared to spend most of your time on the couch? When it comes to chronic pain, feeling discomfort with exertion is not a reliable sign that you should stop all activity and movement. Being active can speed recovery. Unless your activity is excessive, your discomfort may have more to do with reduced muscle flexibility, strength, and endurance than with your original injury or source of pain.

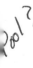

In the case of chronic pain, rest can become atrophy (wasting away of the muscles). But that doesn't mean you should never rest. The key is balance. Contingent rest—resting after motion—is fine. Try looking at rest as a reward for doing good work, not a punishment for getting hurt or ill.

No pain, no gain.   This is the old football coach approach to life. It's right up there with "walk it off." You tell yourself (or someone tells you) to be tough, to work through the pain, to push yourself. But where you often end up pushing yourself is into a pain flare-up.

No pain, no gain is the opposite of "rest is best," but it can be just as bad for you. In some cases, there is absolutely nothing to be gained from pain. Let me give you an example from my own life. To put it mildly, I don't like to go to the dentist, let alone get a shot from the dentist. I don't like needles. So you can imagine how happy I was to hear I needed a dental procedure that usually involves several shots. I decided I could muscle through without Novocain. Bad idea. The dentist was uptight because he could see he was hurting me. And as he worked, the vibrations reverberated against my nerves. They kept reverberating for five days. It was a very long five days.

Several years later, I needed to have the same procedure on another tooth. This time I chose the Novocain. I still didn't like getting needles stuck in my mouth, but I was happy to not feel the procedure. And the next day, I was fine. I gained plenty by choosing the no-pain option.

You must have a pain-prone personality.   There is no such thing as a pain-prone personality, an innate propensity to have chronic illness and pain. Researchers have tried for years to find evidence of such a personality but have always come up short. Some people may view the world in ways that cause them more suffering, but that's not the same as being born with a personality that attracts chronic pain. Part 2 of this book, particularly chapter 8, will help you discover what thoughts, ideas, and behaviors you may be engaging in that are exacerbating and even maintaining your pain problem.

It's all in your head.   Your pain is all in your head in that the brain is the central processing unit of your pain experience. But the Cartesian model of pain (that the degree of pain should be directly tied to the degree of injury) is as outdated as the idea of a flat earth. Pain is much more complicated than René Descartes thought. (See chapter 2 for more about the different models of pain.) Just because a physician can't find a cause for your pain does not mean your pain is imagined. And even a physician who can find a cause does not know your pain. All the X-rays, MRIs, and blood tests in the world can't tell a physician what you feel. Important as it is, a diagnosis is only one piece of a complex puzzle.

The fact that your pain changes also does not mean that your pain is all in your head. If you start getting better without medication or treatment by a physician, that does not mean the pain wasn't real. It means something you are doing is working. Understanding what you did to cause the improvement may be more useful than getting a diagnosis. A diagnosis is very important, but it is not critical to improving your pain experience.

TO SUM UP

The basics of chronic pain are not difficult to understand. But the fact that they are relatively simple does not mean they are unimportant. Quite the contrary. After reading this chapter, you should have a better idea of what constitutes chronic pain, how it differs from acute pain (and why that distinction is important), some of the causes of chronic pain, why self-management is important to your quality of life, and some of the myths and fallacies that can get in the way.

Chapter 2 will continue down this road of education as you learn about various models for understanding chronic pain and take a more comprehensive look at your particular pain.

CHAPTER 2

The Biopsychosocial
Model of Pain

There are many ways to think of pain. In fact, there are as many ways to think about pain as there are people suffering from pain: as a symphony, a dance, a storm. Most, if not all, analogies reflect the idea that pain is a complex dynamic involving more than just pain sensors. Any understanding of pain must also take into consideration gender, heredity, life circumstances, emotions, memory, the reactions of others, and general thoughts about pain.

We all come equipped with the same basic nerve fibers, neurotransmitters, and brain structures, but our pain systems can behave in radically different ways. And you and the people around you must recognize and honor the uniqueness of your pain experience if you hope to ever make any improvement.

It is no revelation that people have different thresholds of pain tolerance. Some people have a very high tolerance for pain; others have virtually no tolerance whatsoever. The level of tolerance must be considered just as important as the extent of the injury. Your perception of your pain *is* your pain.

Our understanding of pain has grown tremendously over the years. Though there is still no definitive way of measuring pain, at least we understand the mechanisms and effects of pain better than our ancestors did.

However, pain management based on the traditional models does not work. Pain is multifaceted and multidimensional, meaning that many factors can affect a person's pain and that pain can be modified through various strategies. This chapter provides a review of pain mechanisms and current thoughts and theories on this complex human experience.

TRADITIONAL PAIN MODELS

Let's take a look at two of the traditional ways of understanding pain: the Cartesian model and the gate-control model.

The Cartesian (Biological) Model of Pain

The explanation for pain that has dominated much of medical history came from the sixteenth-century Western philosopher, physiologist, and mathematician René Descartes. The Cartesian model—essentially a biological model—set forth that anything that could be doubted should be rejected. Under Cartesian thinking, the only useful factor in the pain experience was tissue injury. Tissue injury could be measured; it could be proven. The degree of pain was assumed to be determined by and directly proportional to the degree of injury. Only the physical aspects of pain mattered. Every person with a particular injury was expected to feel and respond exactly the same as every other person with that same injury. In the Cartesian model, tissue injury can be likened to a dial controlling volume; turn up the injury, the tissue damage, and you turn up the pain. But chronic pain has been shown to be much less mechanistic.

The Gate-Control Model of Pain

The Cartesian theory was the firmly accepted way of looking at pain until 1965, when Ronald Melzack, a Canadian psychologist, and Patrick Wall, a British physiologist, put forth the *gate-control* theory of pain. Melzack and Wall (1988) argued that pain signals do not travel simply from the injured tissue to the brain; rather, those signals must go through a gating mechanism in the spinal cord. When the gate is closed, pain is not registered in the brain. When the gate is opened, pain registers. And the gate can be opened or closed by more factors than the signals caused by tissue damage.

The gate-control theory goes beyond a simple focus on the body and takes into account the impact of the mind. Melzack and Wall said that the gate could be opened or closed by emotions, memories, mood, and thoughts. After the signals reach a certain threshold, the brain generates pain sensations. In fact, the brain can register pain even when there is no tissue damage whatsoever (as with phantom pain from amputated limbs). PET scans have shown that parts of the brain light up with pain even when there is no tissue damage.

Despite wide acceptance of the gate-control theory of pain, today's physicians still tend to see pain in Cartesian terms (as a physical process and a sign of tissue damage) because they are trained in Cartesian terms. They know how to look for ruptured disks, fractures, infection, and disease. But when it comes to pain, most physicians get only a few hours of training in pain management, if they get any at all.

THE BIOPSYCHOSOCIAL MODEL: THE FUTURE OF PAIN MANAGEMENT

While there are people who still believe that pain must not be real if a physical cause can't be found, the tide is turning. Unfortunately, some of the people questioning the reality of pain are medical professionals. But the more comprehensive and inclusive biopsychosocial model, pioneered by G. L. Engle (1977), is gaining widespread acceptance as more and more success is reported in its use.

One major drawback to the biological model was that it expected every person with the same injury to experience the same pain. There is no question that the focus of medicine on biological factors improved the quality of our lives. Take medications, for example. Antibiotics give us a powerful weapon against bacterial infections, anti-inflammatory medications reduce swelling and pain, and antihypertensives lower blood pressure. But the biological model did not consider external influences as relevant to disease in general and pain in particular. Anyone who has had a bad day at work and ended up with a headache knows how the two are connected.

Think of the physical and psychological experience of blushing. Blushing is involuntary, but at the same time it is based on an interpretation of an event that requires thoughts. An event occurs, you interpret the event as embarrassing, and your face turns red. Your experience, combined with your interpretation, causes a biological reaction. Similarly, the answers to managing your chronic pain lie in examining what goes on both around you and within you.

Today, our understanding of pain has evolved and broadened. We are beginning to live in the era of the biopsychosocial (BPS) view of pain, which takes into account the biological (physical) influences but also looks at the psychological (emotional) influences and places them in a social (personal) context. The BPS model considers the entire person—body, mind, and environment.

Your pain is real. It is not all in your head. Your head may be part of your problem, but so might your job, your spouse, your doctors, or your medications. Pain perception is influenced by biological, psychological, and social factors that combine and interact in ways unique to you. Understanding the complex nature of your pain is the first step toward improving the quality of your life.

The BPS model of pain makes an important distinction between the physical components of pain and the emotional suffering often associated with chronic pain. How you feel is important, but how you react to those feelings is even more so. How those around you act and react will influence both your feelings and your reactions.

Biological, Psychological, and Social Contributors to Pain

Within the BPS model of pain, many things can influence, maintain, and even worsen your pain. Biological or physical components of pain include:

■ Tissue damage, degenerative changes, and scarring

■ Muscle tension and physical arousal

■ Body mechanics (how you lift and move things)

■ Posture

■ Inflammation

■ Sleep disturbance

■ Fatigue

■ Medications

Psychological or emotional components of pain include:

■ Thoughts, beliefs, and ideas about living with pain (for example, fearing reinjury, struggling with the invisible nature of pain, blaming yourself for having pain, and catastrophizing about pain)

- Anger, frustration, and irritability (*Why me?*)

- Fear

- Depression and anxiety

- Boredom

- Attention to and focus on pain

- Feelings of helplessness and lack of control

Social components of pain include:

- The reactions of your spouse or partner, family, and others to your pain

- Cultural and religious influences

- What you learned about pain as a child

- How you have been treated by doctors and the health care system

- Legal, insurance, and disability systems

Determining the Proportions of Contributing Factors

It helps to try to visualize how much impact the various components have on your life. Some people visualize a glass filled with different colors of sand, each color representing something that affects their pain. Others think of their pain as planets in orbit around them, with the larger planets having a stronger gravitational pull. But for most people, a circle or pizza does the trick.

Imagine that pain is represented by a circle. All the things that contribute to that pain experience are inside this circle. Using the biopsychosocial model, you can estimate how much of your circle is composed of biological and physical factors, how much is psychological or emotional, and what portion is social (influenced by the actions of others). If the circle is a pizza and each category is a slice, how big is each slice?

Sam's Pain Circle

Sam has chronic low back pain from a lifting accident several months ago at work. Sam believes 80 percent of his pain problem is made up of biological and physical factors (such as tissue damage and fatigue). He also feels that 10 percent of his pain experience is related to psychological and emotional factors (such as depression and focusing on his pain). And 10 percent of his pain experience, he believes, is related to his social life, work life, and the frustration he has experienced fighting with the insurance company to get treatment.

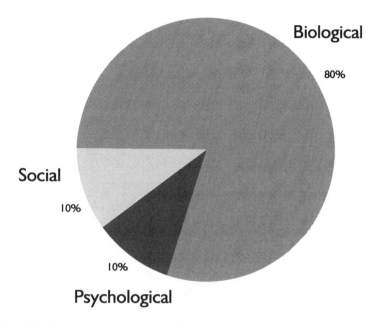

Figure 2.1: Sam's Pain Circle

Betsy's Pain Circle

Betsy, on the other hand, has fibromyalgia and believes that 35 percent of her pain is generated by physical factors, 60 percent is aggravated by stress and frustration, and 5 percent comes from the fact that her friends don't believe her pain is real.

Betsy's allocation is different than Sam's. Everyone is unique when it comes to pain, but this exercise is just as useful across the board.

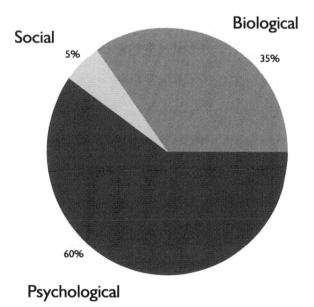

Figure 2.2: Betsy's Pain Circle

EXERCISE 2.1: YOUR PAIN CIRCLE

Now, consider your circle. What percentage of your pain is composed of biological factors? What percentage is psychological or emotional? What portion is social? Make each piece as big or as small as it feels to you. Remember, you can't be wrong, because this is your pain and your experience. You are the expert.

Draw slices in the open circle below to portion out the influence you think these three spheres have on your pain experience.

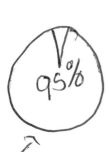

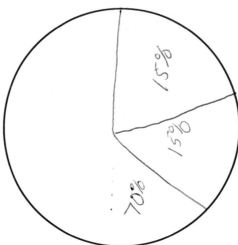

Understanding your pain is crucial to improving your pain experience. Your pain circle is a visual representation of what you believe is contributing to your pain, taking into account your biological (physical), psychological (mental), and social (personal) perspective.

This circle is a snapshot of your unique pain experience. You may want to periodically do the circle exercise again to check your progress as you go through the book. Notice if your slices change size as you learn how the three areas interact.

If you'd like to add another dimension to the circle exercise, redraw your circle to represent how large your pain problem looms in your life: the bigger the size, the bigger the problem. Then, as you work through the book, you can adjust the overall size of your circle along with the relative contributions of the biopsychosocial pieces. Ideally, as you learn to cope more effectively with pain, the overall size of the circle will get smaller and you will have a greater understanding of the role of biological, psychological, and social factors in your pain experience.

TO SUM UP

You should now have a better grasp of the ways pain has been understood in the past. In particular, you should understand the connection between the biological, psychological, and social influences on pain. One factor cannot be viewed without taking into account the others. The circle exercise helps you see your pain in biopsychosocial terms.

Chapter 3 will take a look at where you are in your own personal readiness for change and your intention to change. It will help you examine how willing you are to change, where you may need to change, and where this book fits into that process.

Your Readiness for Change and Intention to Change

The chronic pain experience is like a dance done by two unwilling partners. Your pain is resistant to change because, at least initially, it performs a valuable service for your body. Acute pain is not some malicious entity out to make your life miserable; rather, it is a warning that something is wrong and needs to change. But instead of looking for that change, most people focus on the pain.

When acute pain becomes chronic pain, it turns into a dance of resistance between the person and the pain, and that often leaves people feeling stuck. The message that something is wrong has already been delivered, but the pain continues. And like beginning dance students who only know the tango and therefore try to force all partners into the same rhythm, many people keep trying to force their relationships with pain into one preconceived set of treatments. Those treatments are most likely based on the acute pain model, which aims to stop the pain at all costs.

The problem is that your pain experience is as unique and as personal as your fingerprints. No two people have the same. Your pain is truly yours, and no one but you is as capable of understanding its patterns and nuances. The ebb and flow of your pain and the rhythms of your life must be taken into consideration. A doctor can help, a psychologist can help, nurses and family and friends can all do a world of good, but first you must accept responsibility for the management of your pain. You may always be dancing with the same partner, but at least you can keep from stomping on each other's toes.

YOUR ROLE IN MANAGING YOUR PAIN

The key to an effective arsenal of coping strategies is choice. A wealth of research shows that how well you cope with your pain is based on what you do rather than what is done to you by others. Put simply, most of pain management is what you are willing to do rather than what your doctors can do for you. Remember, it's your pain, not your doctor's. You must be a person—and an active participant in your survival—not just a patient.

Of course, the first thing you need to ask yourself is whether your current coping strategies are working. Odds are, if they were, you wouldn't be reading this book. This workbook will help you take control of your pain by looking at exactly what is contributing to your dance with pain and creating a pain management program tailored to your needs, your lifestyle, and your goals.

You already know you are in pain. You probably know a dozen adjectives for the precise way your pain feels and how it affects you. You've described the pain to doctors, nurses, and relatives so many times you probably don't even think about the words anymore.

People tend to see things in a way that is familiar and stable, comfortable. But maybe it's time to get out of that comfort zone and try something different—not just a new pill or a new exercise, but a new way of thinking about and approaching pain. You can stop being a passive recipient of your chronic pain. Become the manager. When you know your body, your life, and your habits intimately, you can apply a small change for a large payoff. Are you ready for that change?

> If we don't change direction soon, we'll end up where we're going.
>
> —Irwin Corey

Your perception of pain, your medical treatment, your view of personal control, your emotions, and your ideas about experiencing pain can influence not only your pain experience but also your readiness to change and intention to change. And your readiness and intention to change is a critical predictor of your level of engagement in—and success with—a pain self-management plan.

EXERCISE 3.1: EVALUATE YOUR CURRENT COPING STRATEGIES

Changing behavior is not easy, and maintaining that change is even harder. But, as Albert Einstein aptly put it, "Repeating the same behavior expecting different results is insanity." Consequently, you need to look at what you have been doing and identify what has worked and what has not.

What coping strategies do you currently use? Mark any that apply and add your own. Then use a scale of 0 to 10 to rate how well you believe they are working.

		not at all effective								very effective		
☑	Medication	0	1	2	3	④	5	6	7	8	9	10
☑	Rest	0	1	2	3	4	5	⑥	7	8	9	10
☑	Inactivity	0	1	2	③	4	5	6	7	8	9	10
☑	Distraction	0	1	2	3	4	5	6	⑦	8	9	10
☑	Physical therapy	0	1	2	3	4	5	6	7	⑧	9	10
☑	Avoiding activities	⓪	1	2	3	4	5	6	7	8	9	10
☐	_____	0	1	2	3	4	5	6	7	8	9	10

☐ _____   0   1   2   3   4   5   6   7   8   9   10

☐ _____   0   1   2   3   4   5   6   7   8   9   10

If the majority of your coping strategies are not very effective, don't worry. This book is designed to help you learn new ways of coping and build your skills using them. As you fill out your Pain Scorecard, you will see patterns in the factors that help and the factors that hinder your management of your pain.

This simple exercise of separating the wheat from the chaff should help you see that change is possible. Once you begin to look at all you have tried, you will see possibilities. That knowledge, combined with an understanding of all the factors that contribute to your experience of pain, can be a strong potion. But you must be ready and motivated in order to change.

ARE YOU READY TO CHANGE?

The fact that you started reading this book tells me that you are motivated. The fact that you are still reading tells me that you are open to change. You've already started your part of the deal. For my part, I hope this book will motivate you, change how you cope with chronic pain, and improve not only your ability to function and your quality of life but also the quality of your understanding.

The concept of readiness to change was originally described by Prochaska (1984; Prochaska and DiClemente 1983) in his work with problem drinkers. He hypothesized that people respond better to different types of interventions depending on their readiness to adopt new coping skills for drinking behavior. Prominent pain researcher Kerns and his colleagues (1997) adapted Prochaska and DiClemente's stages-of-change model for use with people in pain.

Later in this chapter, I'll discuss each of the stages. First, though, let me point out that readiness to change can be developed. How ready you are now does not necessarily indicate how ready you will be tomorrow, next week, or even next year. Readiness to change is not a constant. Nor is it something you either have or don't have. Motivation can be influenced by your environment, knowledge, skills, and ideas about pain.

EXERCISE 3.2: CONTINUUM OF READINESS

Let's take a look at where you are now. How motivated are you to change? Your readiness to adopt a self-management approach—your commitment to learn adaptive coping skills—can be viewed along a continuum:

_____

not motivated to learn   very motivated to learn
new ways to cope with pain   new ways to cope with pain

Place an X where you currently believe you are on this continuum.

My goal is to motivate you and show you that you can improve your condition. You may not feel willing or ready to try a self-management approach to pain or to stick with a new program. That's normal. Resistance can come from fear, negative expectations, or misinterpretation. But more importantly, once you understand your resistance, you can deal with it and manage it.

 Managing pain is hard work, and you will need to remind yourself why you are learning and practicing these new skills. The simplest way to do so is to review the negative effects pain has on your life.

EXERCISE 3.3: LIST THE NEGATIVES

List below some of the negative aspects of having chronic pain in your life. Think about the physical, social, and psychological aspects of your pain. Consider things like poor sleep, bad mood, and inability to do things you'd like to do.

— work
— home
— activities
— walking
— exercising
— shopping

— apperance.
— restless sleep
— moody
— missing out
— emboressment to family + friends

Keep this list. You can refer back to it when your motivation is low. Remember that you chose to explore new methods of pain management. You must, therefore, believe that it is possible to improve your relationship to your pain. Keep that idea in mind whenever you pull out your list.

LEARNING TO BE ADAPTABLE AND FLEXIBLE

What can you expect from a self-management plan? That depends, of course, on what you want, where you start, and what you are willing to do. The key is to set goals. Some goals you can and should consider are pain reduction, increased strength and activity tolerance, improved concentration, improved sleep, improved mood, reduced fear, and reduced anxiety associated with having pain. Now, isn't that worth working toward?

In this book, you will be asked to do and consider many different things. For example:

■   Are you ready to exercise or change your exercise routine in order to increase strength and endurance and stimulate the release of endorphins for pain control?

■   Are you ready to learn to pace activities and resist either overdoing it or resting too much?

■   Are you ready to challenge your ideas about pain?

- Are you willing to monitor your pain experience using a journal or pain diary?

- Are you willing to modify your sleep habits to reduce pain and fatigue?

- Are you willing to change the way you do chores and recreational activities (like playing golf, driving a car, doing the laundry, or shopping for groceries)?

- Are you a rigid person? Are you willing to reevaluate situations given new facts? Are you still trying to get back to where you were at eighteen? Do you think that's realistic, in terms of pain or anything else? Do you see your life strictly as "before pain" and "after pain," considering one good and the other bad?

If you are willing to change, to learn to be more flexible, to listen to the messages of your body (and this book), and modify how you do things—if you can do that, if you can take that one step—you will improve. Chronic pain is a test of adaptability, flexibility, and your ability to modify your behavior. Those who adapt thrive!

It's easy to lose sight of what's important. Ask yourself if you have lost focus on what is important in terms of your pain problem. Sometimes, it takes flexibility to stay focused.

STAGES OF CHANGE

When Prochaska and DiClemente (1983) developed their readiness-for-change stages, they were working with alcoholics, trying to figure out better ways to help people kick their addiction. Here are the analogous stages of readiness for adopting a self-management approach to chronic pain:

- Expecting a cure

- Not even ready to think about changing

- Open to thinking about changing, but . . .

- Believing change is possible

- Ready to make changes

Expecting a Cure

People in pain often have either a medical or a rehabilitation focus. People with a medical focus are looking for a cure. They want to be fixed and cured and have their pain eliminated for good. They say, *Boy, if I just could get rid of my pain, my life would be better.* People with a rehabilitation focus are also interested in living with less pain, but they are willing to learn and explore new ways to cope with pain based on what they can do for themselves—a self-management approach.

Do you have a medical focus? Consider the following statements. To what extent do you agree or disagree?

My doctors need to take care of me and fix my pain problem.

There are some wonderful doctors out there. All I need to do is find them and they will take care of me.

No matter what people say about learning to live with this pain, I don't think I should have to, especially with all the wonderful things medicine and doctors can do.

There must be a reason for my pain. I know that all I need to do is keep looking and find a doctor who can finally figure it out and fix me.

If you find yourself thinking these thoughts, you are likely in the medical phase. Although this is normal, it does not fit well with a self-management approach to pain. This is not to say that a self-management approach cannot or will not work for you, only that you will need to keep close tabs on your improvements (mental and physical) as you work through this book, because you will need more proof that self-management is working. If you are absolutely positive that no one but a physician can improve your pain experience, then this book may not be useful for you now. Tuck it away and perhaps come back to it sometime in the future if your pain does not diminish.

Not Even Ready to Think About Changing

If you found yourself agreeing with the majority of the above statements, you're not alone. Lots of people think the same way. You likely have the "I'm not a doctor" mind-set. This is the notion that you don't have any information about what may be causing your pain and even less influence over treating it. The "I'm not a doctor" mind-set reflects the belief that you have minimal control of your pain, which can lead you to feel that there is nothing you can do to cope with your pain other than seek the help of doctors. You didn't cause the pain, and you don't have the skills or ability to fix it; only the professionals do. You can't change the pain, and someone else needs to do something to make you feel better. Researchers call this the *precontemplative* stage of change. In this stage, you really aren't even contemplating how to change.

You are not to blame for holding these ideas or beliefs. You have probably had some very positive experiences with doctors in the past that have led to significant improvements with medical problems. Maybe you had a bad toothache, and the dentist was able to fix it and eliminate your pain after filling a cavity. Perhaps you broke your leg while skiing, and after a doctor set your leg and put it in a cast, it was as good as new in a couple of months. Experiences like this can lead you to expect that every pain problem now and in the future will be resolved with treatment from a doctor. So you can see how it's possible to develop the idea that all medical problems can be fixed and cured.

If you hold this belief, you may start to think that it is the doctors' fault that you are still in pain. If they were more competent, you would have gotten better by now. So your energy should be spent looking for the doctor or clinic that can cure your pain. Doing something for yourself is out of the question. After all, it's real, and it's a medical problem, so let them fix it. But chronic pain is often not about fixing, curing, or eliminating so much as it is about coping, managing, and dealing.

Of course, not everybody believes that their doctors are the only ones who can help them with their pain problem. Some people have started to contemplate what they need to do about their own pain. They still may wish their pain could be taken away, but they don't want to have to do much themselves to get rid of the pain.

Common thoughts here include:

People are telling me that I have to learn to live with this pain, but I don't want to have to.

Why should I have to deal with this pain by changing my lifestyle? It's not fair, it's not right, and I don't deserve this.

Open to Thinking About Change, But . . .

Another stage in preparing for change is the "yeah, but" experience. Common thoughts include:

Losing weight and learning better body mechanics probably would help, but that's just way too much to take on.

I tried a new pain medication a couple of months ago, but the side effects were really bad.

I've heard that relaxation exercises can help, but I'm such a tense person, there's no way that would work for me.

A common theme in these statements is *ambivalence*. Being ambivalent means having two opposing ideas, attitudes, or emotions at the same time along with a feeling of uncertainty. People with this mind-set are often under pressure from significant others to pursue a new way of dealing with pain.

"Yeah, but" statements are made by people who are starting to contemplate the need to take a more active role in their pain management. You know you are in pain, and you know you could or should do something to help the situation, but you don't really want to change your life or have to do things differently. You can see what works and what doesn't, but you resist the idea of having to do anything (or do anything more). I worked with one woman several years ago who was very up-front with me during my initial evaluation. She said, "I have done a lot to change my life because of my pain, and I don't want to have to do any more." She was definitely frustrated and angry.

If you find yourself thinking "yeah, but," you are a step closer to being ready for a self-management approach to pain rehabilitation. The way to resolve your ambivalence and move forward is to concentrate on how your life will improve when you master new skills.

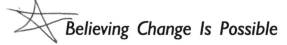

Believing Change Is Possible

In the continuum of readiness, the next step is "I think I can." This stage is characterized by thoughts such as:

I am ready to learn new ways of coping with my pain.

I realize now that it is up to me to do a better job of living with my pain.

This pain may be with me for a long time, so I am willing to adopt new coping strategies.

I realize now that there is no medical cure for my pain, and I want to learn some new ways of coping with it.

People endorsing the "I think I can" notion are like the little engine that could: they have decided to take some action. They are hopeful and empowered. This is the perfect time to identify successful strategies, choose a start date, and make plans.

Ready to Make Changes

People who have the "I think I can" mind-set about their pain readily transition to the "here I go" mind-set once ideas turn to action. This is where real change happens. It's all about learning and doing—learning new coping skills and doing what it takes to improve quality of life. Thoughts at this stage include:

I have learned and am learning some good ways to keep my pain problem from interfering with my life.

I can get on with the business of living despite my pain.

Pain management is no longer a white-knuckle, day-to-day battle. At this point, you have modified your life to a degree that management of pain is a natural part of the day. You have the skills to manage the pain and the confidence to keep those skills going. To keep momentum, you need to identify precisely what actions, circumstances, or thoughts trigger a pain flare-up so that you can defuse them when they come along. A real commitment to change has occurred, and it may even be one that can be shared by other people. Significant others may show a willingness to change along with you—either as a show of support or because your pain is affecting them, too.

TAKING ACTION!

Now you have a handle on where you are in your readiness to change. But information alone does not lead to change. Knowledge is wonderful. It is the grease that will make it easier to keep going once the train is in motion, but it does not start the train moving. Information must be coupled with action. You may just be inspired to take action, or there may be an outside impetus.

Hitting bottom (however you might define that) may be the push that gets you started. But better is when you recognize that your life would be easier with some help. Don't be afraid to get connected with people who have experience helping others: physicians, psychologists with experience in pain, physical therapists, occupational therapists, nurses, case managers. Find people to help keep your train going strong.

TO SUM UP

You should now understand that change is not instantaneous; rather, it is a gradual process. And there is a continuum of readiness to change and intention to change. Knowing where you are on that continuum is your first step. You need to know where you are before you start so that you know what direction to set out in.

Chapter 4 will continue along the path of education and self-awareness, exploring how you rate your pain and how you measure it. From here, you can set goals that you can achieve and that will improve your quality of life.

CHAPTER 4

Rating Pain, Monitoring Flare-Ups, and Setting Goals

Self-knowledge, or understanding your pain experience, is the foundation upon which a self-management program for pain is built. The cornerstone of understanding your pain experience is understanding your pain. The raw material of understanding your pain is using a pain scale. In this chapter, I'll walk you through rating your pain, understanding your pain flare-ups, and setting goals about pain management.

RATING YOUR PAIN

The first things a physician learns in medical school are the four vital signs: pulse, respiration, blood pressure, and temperature. But there is a fifth, all-important vital sign: pain.

Being able to estimate and rate your pain allows you to track changes in your pain experience. Since one of the primary goals of the self-management approach is to reduce the overall intensity of your pain, it is important to use a consistent technique for measuring your pain.

The Pain Intensity Scale

Pain is personal, subjective, and unique to you. There is no perfect measurement, but a good pain scale allows you to rate your pain and see progress over time. The pain intensity scale below is particularly useful because it includes descriptive phrases to clarify what each range of numbers means. Some researchers believe that this type of combination scale is least affected by gender and ethnic differences in describing pain. Not everyone sees a 3 on a scale of 0 to 10 as the same. But most people can agree on what "functional" means if it's defined as "You are aware of pain, and your daily life is affected somewhat, but the impact on your life is minimal." There is less room for variation with a more detailed description.

Use this scale throughout the book so you have a <u>consistent standard</u> to compare any changes that occur as you do the exercises and implement the suggestions in this book.

	Mild	**Moderate**	**Severe**	
0	1 2 3	4 5 6 7	8 9	10
No Pain	**Functional**	**Uncomfortable**	**Severe**	**Unbearable**
	■ you are aware of pain ■ your daily life is affected somewhat ■ the impact on your life is minimal	■ it's hard to move ■ you have difficulty concentrating ■ the pain interferes with activities of living	■ you cannot leave home ■ you have difficulty doing anything	■ the pain is out of control ■ you find it necessary to seek medical care

EXERCISE 4.1: RATE YOUR CURRENT PAIN

Using the 0 to 10 scale, estimate your pain over the past twenty-four hours.

What was your pain at its average? _5/6_

Understanding Improvement in Scores

Scores of 0 to 3, 4 to 7, and 8 to 10 appear to be distinct categories that differentiate people suffering from chronic pain. People who score in the same range tend to resemble each other in their level of daily functioning, and levels of functioning vary consistently between groups. In other words, people tend to fall into groups that share similar characteristics. People who average scores of 0 to 3 will have more in common with each other than they will with people who score 4 or higher. People who average scores of 4 to 7 will have more in common with each other than with people who score in the upper range.

If your pain level is 1 to 4, a decrease in pain of just one point corresponds to a clinically meaningful improvement in functioning. That means that if you move from a score of 3 to 2, it's a big deal. But if your pain is rated as 5 to 10, a two-point decrease is necessary for a meaningful improvement. Moving from 7 to 6 is good, but moving from 7 to 5 is great.

The effectiveness of your individualized self-management program can be evaluated not only in terms of average pain reductions (change in numbers), but also in terms of whether your pain is reduced from one category of pain intensity to another (for example, from uncomfortable to functional or from severe to uncomfortable). This is what we are working for: a change in overall intensity and a change in category.

Comparing Scores

Rating your pain with one number at one time in the day may not be as accurate as taking several measures across the day or even the week. This is certainly true if your pain fluctuates a lot. Also, moderate pain experienced all or almost all of the time may be more disabling than severe pain experienced intermittently. For this reason, it can be helpful to take three readings of your pain (worst, average, and least) for a given day. Using the 0 to 10 point scale and taking three separate readings yields a range from 0 to 30 for that day.

Let's look at two hypothetical people and their pain scores. For Thursday, Mary rated her worst pain a 9, her least pain a 5, and her average pain a 7. Her total is 21 points for the day. Tom, on the other hand, rated his worst pain at an 8 and his lowest pain a 6, with an average of 7. His total score was also 21. Mary and Tom both have the same total score and the same average, but their pain experience is very different. Mary had a higher "worst" score and a lower "least" score. Tom's pain varied less over the course of the day. People experience pain differently, and simply comparing one set of scores between people does not give the full picture. What matters is the changes that a single person experiences over time.

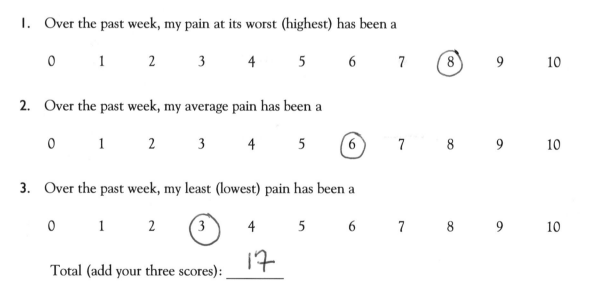

EXERCISE 4.2: RATE YOUR PAIN OVER THE PAST WEEK

Use the 0 to 10 pain intensity scale to complete the following statements.

1. Over the past week, my pain at its worst (highest) has been a

    0   1   2   3   4   5   6   7   (8)   9   10

2. Over the past week, my average pain has been a

    0   1   2   3   4   5   (6)   7   8   9   10

3. Over the past week, my least (lowest) pain has been a

    0   1   2   (3)   4   5   6   7   8   9   10

    Total (add your three scores): ___17___

    Your total score should be between 0 and 30.

Now, go to the Pain Scorecard at the back of this book and enter your score. Notice what level you scored: one (minimal impact), two (moderate impact), or three (significant negative impact). For many of the exercises in this book, you'll transfer your results to the Pain Scorecard. The ultimate goal is to help you tailor your treatment to your particular level.

TRACKING YOUR PAIN

Even if you feel that you know your pain inside and out, tracking your pain over time and monitoring how it changes is important. Many people will swear up and down that they know all they need to know about when their pain worsens and when it gets better, but when they actually start writing down when and under what circumstances their pain worsens, they learn some interesting new things.

As a way to really get to know more about your unique pain experience, keep a Discovery Journal and a Daily Activity and Pain Level Chart for one week. You may want to photocopy these pages or go to my Web site (www.PainCareWorkbook.com), where you can download the worksheets.

EXERCISE 4.3: DISCOVERY JOURNAL

Date and day: _____

(For pain intensity, mood, and energy level, use a 0 to 10 scale, with 0 being the lowest and 10 being the highest.)

Pain intensity ratings	Medication:	Dosage:	Time:	Previous Night's Sleep
Morning 0 1 2 3 ④ 5 6 7 8 9 10	tramadol	_____	6:00	Time lights out: 11:30 Minutes till sleep: 5 Time up: 5:00
Afternoon 0 1 ② 3 4 5 6 7 8 9 10	~~tramadol~~	_____	forgot	Number of interruptions: 4 Total hours slept: 5½ Time spent in bed: 5½
Evening 0 1 2 ③ 4 5 6 7 8 9 10	_____	_____	_____	How rested upon awakening (0–10)? 5 Sleep medications used? yes (no)

Total pain score: _____

Depression: ____   **Anger/frustration:** ____   **Anxiety/fear:** ____   **Total mood score:** ____

Energy Level: _____

Coping Strategies Used: _____

Notes: _____

Reviewing your week's worth of Daily Activity and Pain Level Charts, notice whether your activity levels have anything to do with your pain levels. When are you most in pain? What time of the day? Does your pain increase over the course of the day? When is it at its least? Do increases in activity levels influence your pain levels? You will use the information from this chart to understand your pain flare-ups later in this chapter. Likewise, the Discovery Journal gives you valuable information about how your level of pain is related to mood, sleep, medication, and sense of control over pain. Don't worry if you don't feel ready to sort out how these factors are related. For now, you're just gathering information. As you progress through the book, I'll guide you in taking a closer look at each of these factors.

By simply monitoring your pain experience for one week, an interesting thing will likely happen: your pain experience will change. Yes, it will change. Numerous studies have shown that simply monitoring a behavior will actually change it. Then we need to explore how to make that change work for you. That is what lies in the rest of this book.

PAIN CYCLES AND THE NEGATIVE FEEDBACK LOOP

Chronic pain can lead to changes in your life and the way you do things. It can set up a series of negative experiences that can then aggravate the pain that started the process. Negative pain cycles can spin out of control, leaving you feeling helpless. Helplessness leads to frustration and anger. Increased frustration and anger can set the stage for you to overdo activities and aggravate your already present pain. These vicious, self-perpetuating cycles work to maintain your pain problem. In gaining insight into how your behaviors are contributing to your pain cycles, you can gain more control over your pain.

Biopsychosocial Components of the Pain Cycle

Using the biopsychosocial model, let's look at how each component of the chronic pain experience can feed the negative cycles of pain.

Biological Components

Biological components of chronic pain can cause more pain in the following ways:

- Pain can disturb your sleep, which can lead to more pain.

- Pain can lead to physical muscular tension (bracing yourself, guarding a painful area, or limping), which can cause more pain.

- Pain can lead to decreased activity, followed by overactivity to make up for lost time, which can lead to more pain.

- Pain can lead to inactivity, which can lead to atrophy, which can lead to more pain.

- Pain can make it difficult for you to eat well, and a poor diet can deplete your energy, which can lead to fatigue and to more pain.

- Pain can make you feel tired, which can lead to inactivity, which can lead to atrophy and more pain.

EXERCISE 4.4: DAILY ACTIVITY AND PAIN LEVEL CHART

On the graph below, draw a solid line that represents your level of physical activity over the course of the day, with 0 being not at all active and 10 being very active. Then, using a different color pen or a dotted line instead of a solid line, draw a line that represents your pain level over the course of the day.

Date: _____   Day: _____

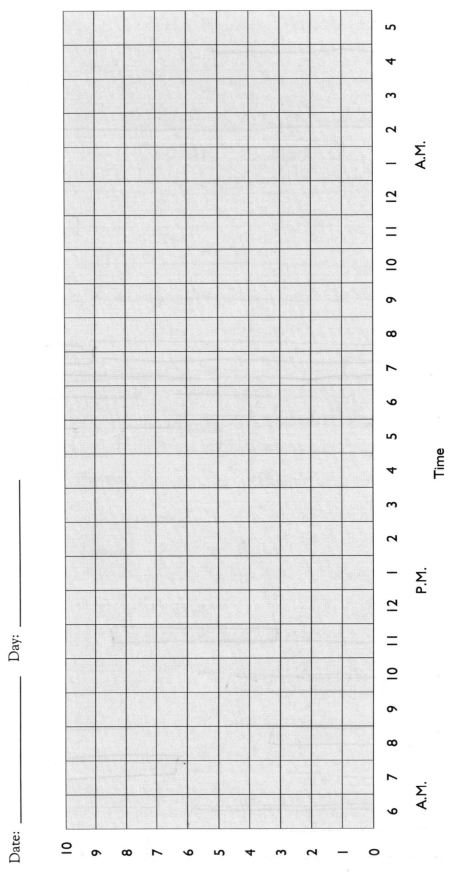

Psychological Components

■ Pain can cause you to feel depressed, which can lead to inactivity, which can lead to more pain.

■ Pain can lead to anxiety, which can cause more pain.

■ Pain can lead to anger, which can lead to more pain.

■ Pain can bring up negative, unproductive thoughts, which can lead to more pain.

■ Pain can lead you to focus on your pain, which can lead you to notice more pain.

■ Pain can make you feel helpless, which can increase your sense of pain.

■ Pain can make you feel bored, which can lead to more pain.

Social Components

Pain can isolate you from other people, which can lead to more pain.

Pain can draw negative attention from others, which can lead to more pain.

Pain can lead you to feel that others don't understand you or don't believe you, which can lead to more pain.

Breaking Pain Cycles

It's important to note that intervening at any part of the pain cycle can be effective in altering the overall cycle. Negative pain cycles can cross the biopsychosocial domain, with factors from each domain playing a role in your pain experience. Reduce tension and muscular bracing, and you can reduce pain. Alter pain, and sleep may improve. Examining your specific pain cycles can be an important step in regaining control of your life.

PAIN FLARE-UPS

One way to gain a better understanding of your unique pain experience is to consider your pain in terms of a series of changes in intensity over time. Learning that a pain flare-up has a beginning, middle, and end is important. Pain levels are never constant, but vary continuously. Knowing how your pain changes can help you predict, prepare for, and reduce the intensity of your pain.

Finding clues as to what makes your pain worse will make your pain more predictable and give you a greater sense of control. Breaking down the various parts of your pain experience into manageable components—and determining better coping methods for each component—begins with an understanding of the concept of a pain flare-up.

What Is a Pain Flare-Up?

Flare-ups aren't random. Your actions, mood, and interactions with others can all increase your chances of experiencing a flare-up at any given time. You probably already knew some of your high-risk situations before you opened the book. You've probably noticed behaviors, times of day, and moods that send you into a flare-up. But have you thought all the way through a flare-up?

Consider that there is a beginning, middle, and end to each pain flare-up. By breaking your pain down into steps, phases, or flare-ups, you can understand it better and bring some predictability to the experience. Pain is at its most disturbing and uncomfortable when it comes out of the blue and seems to last forever. When you understand the trajectory of your pain flare-ups, you gain a sense of control over your pain. Best of all, you can learn to stop pain spirals midspin.

Figure 4.1 shows a typical pain flare-up. Perhaps it starts at a relatively low level of discomfort (1 on a scale of 0 to 10) and is almost imperceptible. This is your *pain threshold*, the point where you first begin to feel the pain. But over a short period of time, it lets you know it is there. The pain gradually gets worse until it reaches its peak (in this example, a 9.5). This is your *tolerance limit*, the point where you have difficulty tolerating the pain. The interesting thing about chronic pain, though, is that it never stays at a 9.5 all the time. It gradually comes back down to the level that you have become accustomed to—whatever that is for you. So what you see is a flare-up with a beginning, middle, and end.

Your goal is to be able to identify the unique triggers that start your pain flare-ups, employ new coping strategies early on in each flare-up, and reduce the frequency, intensity, and duration of your flare-ups. Figure 4.2 shows the trajectory of a pain flare-up with and without adaptive coping strategies.

When you can create a sense of predictability and learn what things make your pain worse, you can begin to make it better. But in order to make that change for the better, you need to look at more than one flare-up. Figure 4.3 shows a graph for someone who had five flare-ups over the course of seven days.

On Monday, this person's pain level started to get bad, rising to a 5. It worsened on Tuesday, reaching an 8. Wednesday was a better day, and the pain went back down to a 3. On Thursday, the pain gradually increased, until late that night it hit a 9. On Friday, the pain first diminished but then rose to a 5 before falling to a low of 2. Saturday saw a bad pain flare-up reaching an 8. Sunday was a good day, and the pain dropped to a low of 2.

EXERCISE 4.5: GRAPH YOUR FLARE-UPS

For each of the next fourteen weeks, place a dot on the graph representing your number of pain flare-ups for that week. Then draw a line connecting the dots.

This graph will help you monitor your flare-ups and give you a *baseline*, a measure of the frequency of your pain flare-ups before you start implementing the treatment suggestions in this workbook. You'll then be able to see any improvements that come from using these new strategies.

Understanding Factors That Influence Flare-Ups

The importance of the concept of a pain flare-up is that there are *triggers*: events or influences that initiate and launch the flare-up. Some triggers are fairly obvious (such as overdoing some activity or

Pain Flare-up

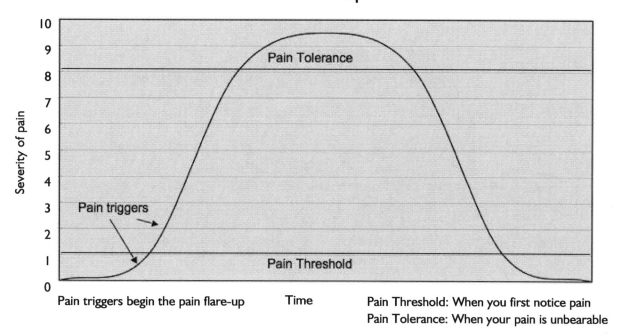

Pain triggers begin the pain flare-up   Time   Pain Threshold: When you first notice pain
Pain Tolerance: When your pain is unbearable

Figure 4.1: Pain Flare-Up

Original Pain Flare-up compared to Modified Pain Flare-up following Adaptive Coping

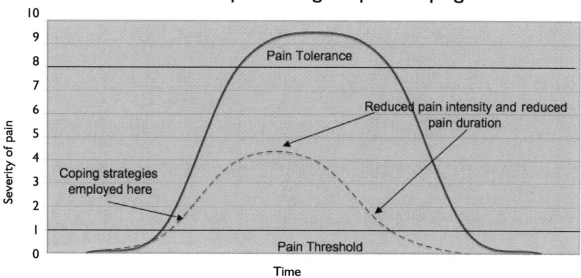

Figure 4.2: Original Pain Flare-Up Compared to Pain Flare-Up with Adaptive Coping

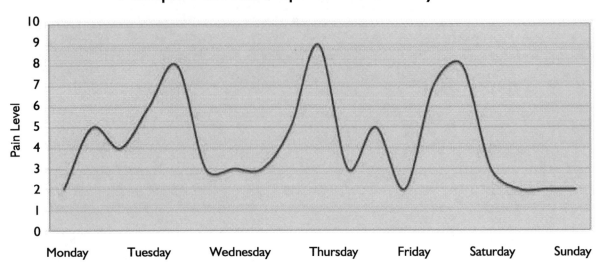

Figure 4.3: Multiple Pain Flare-Ups Over Seven Days

FLARE-UP TRACKING FORM

Goal is to reduce the number of pain flare-ups over time.

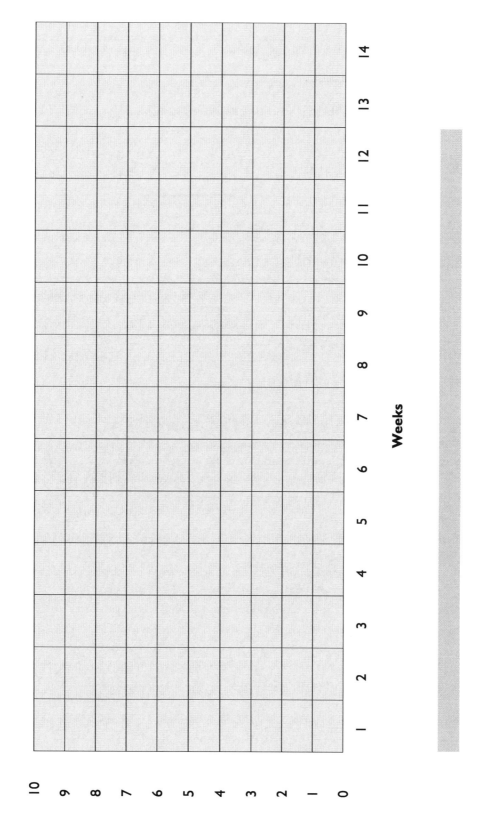

chore, or being under a lot of stress), and some may be very subtle (such as your diet, or your ideas and thoughts about having pain.) As you work through this book, you will become much better at recognizing and avoiding your personal triggers.

These triggers may be biological, psychological, or social. Each domain includes some triggers you can control and some you can't. Whether your triggers are obvious or not, it will be helpful to realize the sheer variety of factors that can influence your pain.

Physical factors that can make your pain worse include the extent of your injury, the readiness of your nervous system to send pain signals, and excessive activity levels. Psychological or emotional factors that can worsen your pain include depression, anxiety, anger, tension, and worry; attention to the pain; boredom; and counterproductive ideas about pain. Social factors that can worsen your pain include the way pain was expressed and talked about in your family, cultural influences, the context of your pain situation, and other people asking you about your pain.

Luckily, there is an equally large realm of factors that can counteract pain. Like triggers, these fall into the physical, psychological, and social domains. Physical factors that can shut down pain include medication, counterstimulation (heat, massage, transcutaneous electrical nerve stimulation, or acupuncture), and moderate exercise. Psychological and emotional factors include relaxation, rest, positive emotions, healthy ideas about pain, a sense of being involved in life activities, and distraction. Social factors that can reduce pain include doing something fun, being treated as normal by your friends, and engaging yourself in work or other purposeful pursuits.

Understanding Which Factors You Can Control

Knowing what factors you can control and what factors you can't allows you to focus your energy, time, and thoughts where they will do the most good. If you have a condition that has no cure, focusing on a cure may be counterproductive. If you know cold weather exacerbates your pain, it may be counterproductive for you to bemoan a snowy day—unless, of course, you are willing to move to a warmer climate. But if you know your pain increases when you run, you can choose when or if you run. If you know your pain increases when you are bored, you can keep yourself busy.

Some common triggers that are not under your control include the weather, things other people do or say to you, "the system" (medical, legal, and insurance establishments), illness, injury, or how your body heals. Common triggers that are under your control include how you react to others, the quantity and quality of sleep you get, medications you use or don't use, your activity level, your emotions, the level of tension you experience, your attitudes, your ideas, your beliefs, how assertive you are, how perfectionistic you are, and how much social contact you have with family and friends.

Through the course of this book, through the exercises and your Pain Scorecard, you will see what elements you control and to what extent you control them. You will be able to stop spinning your wheels trying to change factors outside your realm of influence, leaving you more energy to power up the hills that are currently slowing you down. Throughout this book, I'll suggest ways to use your strengths and challenges to better your quality of life through specific treatment recommendations based on your scores.

Lessons from Flare-Ups

Pain flare-ups are often inevitable. I'd love to say otherwise, but experience has shown me that when it comes to chronic pain, a goal of improvement is more realistic than a goal of cure. But don't discount the power of improvement. Improvement means feeling better. Reducing the overall frequency, intensity, and duration of your pain is a major accomplishment and improvement.

Change in your flare-ups is possible. Keep in mind that flare-ups aren't all the same. Some are smaller or less extreme; others are huge and life altering. Some are a nuisance; others are overwhelming. A minor pain flare-up is a warning. With the right tools, you can stop minor flare-ups from spiraling out of control. Rather than assuming that an increase in pain is the beginning of a full-blown incident, try reframing the experience. Stop your habitual thoughts that predict catastrophe at the first sign of pain, and apply more productive thoughts. A minor flare-up need not be a catastrophe. Rather, it can be an opportunity to use all you've learned to take control and stop the pain in its tracks.

Consider the importance of timing your use of coping strategies. Don't wait to employ the coping strategy until your pain is at its peak. The time to intervene is when your pain is first starting to increase, at the beginning of the flare-up, not when you are already feeling overwhelmed.

Just think how much more in charge you will feel (and, indeed, be) if you recognize an increase in pain right away and stop it from getting worse. You will feel more competent. And just that—feeling you can handle your pain experience—reduces the likelihood of a major flare-up. When you are in pain and encounter one of your potential triggers, you will choose responses to the pain and to the risk of increased pain based on how you think you will be able to cope. Knowing you can cope, knowing you have the knowledge and tools to take control, decreases the intensity of your flare-up. This pattern—minor flare-up, sense of competence, use of adaptive tools, decrease in the intensity of the pain—changes how you think about your pain. Changing how you think about your pain changes your pain.

Keep in mind that your high-risk situations may be someone else's comfort zone. Some people are hugely affected by their level of activity—overdoing it always sends them into a flare-up—while others have flare-ups only when they're bored or stressed. Still others are fine with single risks, but when the risks combine—they are stressed, and it's the end of the day—they can expect increased pain.

There also may be signs associated with an impending flare-up. Do you notice certain behavior signs preceding an increase in pain: limping, holding your head, sighing? Or maybe the sign is in your head: thoughts of how bad your pain is, how it will never be better, how anything you do will only make it worse. Maybe it's mood: depression, loneliness, anger.

Don't worry if you don't know all the answers right now. We are just getting started. Part 2 will offer a multitude of exercises to help you better understand your pain, your response to pain, and what might improve your experience.

EXERCISE 4.6: PAIN FLARE-UP RECORD

Keeping a record of the details of your flare-ups will help you understand the anatomy of your pain. This worksheet covers the biopsychosocial factors that have been found to frequently contribute to pain flare-ups. Use the worksheet to begin to analyze your next pain flare-ups. The form is also available as part of the Pain Care Kit on my Web site (www.PainCareWorkbook.com).

Pain Flare-Up Record

Complete this worksheet for each separate episode of pain you have.

Date started: _____ Time started: _____ A.M./P.M. Time subsided: _____ A.M./P.M.

Situation (What happened before your pain started?)

_____

_____

Pain Rating

Circle the range of numbers that represents your pain during this flare-up.

no pain   unbearable
  0   1   2   3   4   5   6   7   8   9   10

Depression: _____ **Anxiety/Fear:** _____ **Anger/Frustration:** _____ **Other emotion:** _____
(rate each 0 to 10, with 0 being none and 10 being the worst)

What are the triggers that contributed to this flare-up? Check those that apply and circle the one you perceive as the most important trigger.

Biological and Physical Triggers

☐   Muscle tension, tightness, being keyed up

☐   Poor body mechanics (how you lift and move things)

☐   Poor posture

☐   Inflammation

☐   Overdoing it, pushing too hard

☐   Scar tissue, nerve damage, disk damage

☐   Sleep disturbance

☐   Fatigue

☐   Weather changes (change in temperature or barometric pressure)

Psychological Triggers (ideas and thoughts)

☐   *My doctors have missed something.*

☐   *I need more medications.*

☐   *I need more diagnostic testing.*

☐   *I cannot stop the pain.*

- ☐ *This is awful.*

- ☐ *This pain is out of control.*

- ☐ *I can't get on with the business of living.*

- ☐ *I need to rest so I don't make my pain worse.*

- ☐ *I should be careful what I do physically, since I could reinjure myself.*

- ☐ *I give up. Nothing further can be done to eliminate my pain.*

- ☐ *I should be able to control the pain much better than I do.*

- ☐ *I must be doing something wrong that keeps this pain going on and on.*

- ☐ *I shouldn't let the pain bother me.*

- ☐ *I deserve better than to have chronic pain.*

- ☐ *I shouldn't have to suffer with this pain.*

- ☐ *It isn't right that I'm experiencing chronic pain.*

- ☐ *I will never enjoy life again with this pain.*

- ☐ *I will never be completely happy as long as I have this pain.*

- ☐ *My life will never be fulfilling as long as I have this pain.*

Social triggers

- ☐ Being asked to do too much

- ☐ Feeling others aren't helping enough

- ☐ Feeling others don't believe the pain is real

- ☐ Feeling obliged to prove to others that the pain is real

What did I do before the flare-up?

_____

What did I do during this flare-up?

_____

What did I do after this flare-up?

_____

Daniel's Flare-Up Record

Here is what a completed worksheet looked like for Daniel, a thirty-seven-year-old carpenter injured on the job.

DANIEL'S PAIN FLARE-UP RECORD

Complete this worksheet for each separate episode of pain you have.

Date started: _4/12/05_ Time started: _8:30_ (A.M)/P.M.   Time subsided: _9:00_ (A.M)/P.M.

Situation (What happened before your pain started?)

Had to move some boxes in the garage, but no one was around to help me.

Pain Rating

Circle the range of numbers that represents your pain during this flare-up.

no pain   unbearable
 0   1   2   3   4   (5   6   7   8)   9   10

Depression: _7_ **Anxiety/Fear:** _6_ **Anger/Frustration:** _9_ **Other emotion:** _____
(rate each 0 to 10, with 0 being none and 10 being the worst)

What are the triggers that contributed to this flare-up? Check those that apply and circle the one in each section you perceive as the most important trigger.

Biological and physical triggers

☐   Muscle tension, tightness, being keyed up

☑   Poor body mechanics (how you lift and move things)

☐   Poor posture

☐   Inflammation

☐   Overdoing it, pushing too hard

☐   Scar tissue, nerve damage, disk damage

☑   (Sleep disturbance)

☑   Fatigue

☐   Weather changes (change in temperature or barometric pressure)

Psychological triggers (ideas and thoughts)

☐   *My doctors have missed something.*

☑   *I need more medications.*

☐   *I need more diagnostic testing.*

☐   *I cannot stop the pain.*

☐   *This is awful.*

☑   *This pain is out of control.*

☐   *I can't get on with the business of living.*

☐   *I need to rest so I don't make my pain worse.*

☐   *I should be careful what I do physically, since I could reinjure myself.*

☐   *I give up. Nothing further can be done to eliminate my pain.*

☐   *I should be able to control the pain much better than I do.*

☑   *I must be doing something wrong that keeps this pain going on and on.*

☐   *I shouldn't let the pain bother me.*

☑   *I deserve better than to have chronic pain.*

☐   *I shouldn't have to suffer with this pain.*

☐   *It isn't right that I'm experiencing chronic pain.*

☐   *I will never enjoy life again with this pain.*

☐   *I will never be completely happy as long as I have this pain.*

☑   *My life will never be fulfilling as long as I have this pain.*

Social triggers

☐   Being asked to do too much

☑   Feeling others aren't helping enough

☐   Feeling others don't believe the pain is real

☐   Feeling obliged to prove to others that the pain is real

What did I do before the flare-up?

I had not slept well the night before, and then I moved some boxes.

What did I do during this flare-up?

I lay down and rested.

What did I do after this flare-up?

I thought that I would never get over this pain and felt sorry for myself because no one was helping me.

GOALS AND PAIN MANAGEMENT

If you don't know where you want to go, your odds of getting there are slim. Goals are the road map to improving your pain experience. They are not only the destination but the directions. Without goals, you move aimlessly through life without purpose.

Spending your life wishing you felt better won't get you anywhere. But taking the time to decide exactly what feeling better means to you gives you a destination you can work toward. And the directions to get to feeling better will be different depending on the destination. For example, if feeling better means being able to walk a mile without a flare-up, you can work on slowly increasing your activity at a pace that does not increase your pain. But if feeling better means being able to sleep six hours without interruptions, then it really won't matter much how far you walk. The steps need to match the goals. The goals determine the steps.

The High Five of Goal Setting

The first step is to set realistic goals for pain management. Once you have set realistic goals, you can experiment to see which suggestions in this book improve your ability to handle the pain. Strong, achievable goals have five characteristics. They are meaningful, realistic, flexible, positive, and written. Let's look at the characteristics one by one.

Meaningful

Your goals should be meaningful and important to you. They shouldn't be what you think you should want or what you think your doctor, your wife, or your boss might want. How do *you* want to be different? What do you want to change? Are there particular symptoms you would like to target? Your goals should reflect what you would most like to change about your pain experience.

Be specific. Write your goals in a way that includes both the destination and the directions. Goals should also be concrete, consisting of actions, not whims. For example, deciding to improve your ability to cope with pain by increasing your physical activities—such as walking for ten minutes three times a week—is concrete and specific, and it tells you what you need to do.

Realistic

Your goals need to be within your ability. Failure breeds depression, and depression breeds pain. Make your goals challenging but achievable. You may not be able to end your pain, but you can manage it. You may not be able to get your old life back, but you can have a quality of life that brings you joy. Decide what symptoms you most want to change and what would be a significant degree of change. Can you realistically achieve the goal? How confident are you that you can achieve it? You could ask yourself, *On a scale of 0 percent to 100 percent, how confident am I that I can achieve this goal?* The more confident you are, the more likely you will reach your goal.

Flexible

Avoid black-and-white, all-or-nothing thinking. Examine your expectations as you make your goals, and see if you are limiting yourself by being rigid or inflexible. Wanting to get all the laundry done in one day may be too much physically if four loads have piled up. Breaking this down to two loads over two days is an example of flexibility.

Positive

Concentrate on things you want to add to your life, not things you want to subtract or get rid of. Talk about what you will do, not what you will stop or try not to have. Think in terms of "increase" and "gain" rather than "decrease" and "lose."

Written

Write down your goals. Give them the force and permanence of ink. Then post them somewhere you can see them often.

Setting Effective Goals

"I don't want to be depressed" is not the best worded goal. Not only is it negative, but it also offers no solutions to the problem—it doesn't tell you what to do. "I will increase pleasant activities, such as going to visit a friend, to help improve my mood" is a much more effective goal statement because it is positive and tells you what to do. "I will go to one movie per week" may be concrete, meaningful, and positive, but is it realistic? If sitting for two hours triggers your pain, movies could be tough. So you might scratch that goal. But wait, who says seeing a movie means sitting for two hours? Be flexible. Maybe you could stand at the back of the theater or pick a short movie. In the next exercise in this chapter, I'll help you think through the five characteristics and write down some meaningful, concrete, specific, and flexible goals that you can use to start your pain self-management program.

The following are some examples of the strongest and most effective goals I've seen in my practice, paired with vague and weak goals that tried to accomplish the same thing.

Physical or Biological Goals

Goal: Lose weight to reduce pressure on back and spine

Effective goal statement: "I will increase my physical activity level by walking ten minutes a day three days a week to reduce my weight."

Ineffective goal statement: "I want to get rid of this spare tire around my waist."

Goal: Get a better night's sleep

Effective goal statement: "I will go to bed around the same time every night and get up around the same time every morning to get back into a consistent sleep rhythm."

Ineffective goal statement: "I want to have fewer interruptions in my sleep."

Goal: Reduce pain

Effective goal statement: "I will pace my activities better, spreading them out over the course of the day, to reduce my chances of having a pain flare-up."

Ineffective goal statement: "I want to get rid of my pain."

Psychological or Emotional Goals

Goal: Improve my mood

Effective goal statement: "I will lift my mood by going to the library once a week."

Ineffective goal statement: "I don't want to feel depressed anymore."

Goal: Feel more empowered to improve my pain experience

Effective goal statement: "I will do some research on reputable Web sites in order to understand my diagnosis better."

Ineffective goal statement: "I don't want to feel so overwhelmed."

Social Goals

Goal: Reconnect with my partner

Effective goal statement: "I will spend fifteen minutes each day asking questions about my partner's day."

Ineffective goal statement: "I want to fight less with my partner because of my pain."

Goal: Engage in some form of work

Effective goal statement: "I will spend one hour a week at the local blood bank helping with paperwork and filing."

Ineffective goal statement: "I want to help people and feel like I am contributing to the welfare of others."

Other common pain management goals include using pacing to gradually increase movement, improving body mechanics and posture, seeking accurate information about pain management, learning relaxation skills such as diaphragmatic breathing and visualization, and increasing pleasant activities.

EXERCISE 4.7: ESTABLISH YOUR GOALS

Think of ways you would like to be different, symptoms you would like to improve, and ways you want to improve in coping with your pain. Jot down as many ideas as you want, then decide on the top five. Then work through the three parts of goal setting for each.

1. Write a rough draft of your goal.

I will _increase my mobility by using my sit & be fit videos 3-4 times a week._

2. Evaluate your goal.

How important is it that you achieve this goal, and why?   10
Because I want to be more active for my self, kids & job.

Does this goal tell you what to do in real, specific, and positive steps?

yes

Is it realistic given your current situation and circumstances?

yes

On a scale of 0 percent to 100 percent, how confident are you that you can achieve this goal?

90%

How will you know when you have reached your goal?
When I have completed 21 wks in a row
of 3/4 times a week.

3. Write down the final version of your goal.

Make sure it is meaningful, realistic, specific, achievable, flexible, and positive. There is space below for your top five goals.

1. Increase mobility

2. Lose weight

3. lower blood sugar

4. increase social activities

5. Start physical therapy

Now that you've set some goals, it's time to pick a goal and start working toward it.

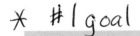
* #1 goal

EXERCISE 4.8: WHAT HAPPENS WHEN YOU WORK TOWARD YOUR GOAL?

Choose a goal from your top five and begin to implement the steps of working toward it. On the Flare-Up Tracking Form, which you started in exercise 4.5, mark the point when you began working toward this goal.

Make sure you <u>change only one part of your daily routine at a time</u>, so you can tell what actually makes the difference. Try to remain consistent in your approach. That is, stick with what you have decided to do.

Once you've completed the Flare-Up Tracking Form, ask yourself these questions:

How has the number of flare-ups per week changed as you've implemented steps toward your goal?

Have you noticed any change in your mood since you started working toward this goal?

Has there been any change in your sleep patterns or the quality of your sleep?

Have you noticed any change in your thoughts or ideas about pain?

Has there been any change in your interactions with friends or family?

TO SUM UP

Your diagnosis is important. Your understanding of your diagnosis is even more so. A good pain self-management program must begin with a real understanding of the problem. This understanding should be shared by your doctors, family, and friends—anyone who can be part of your pain management team. You are the team leader, so it is your job to make sure everyone is starting on the same page, with the same point of reference and with the same goals in mind.

CHAPTER 5

Understanding Your Diagnosis

Knowing what is causing your pain is of the utmost importance in your pain self-management program. Not only do you need to know this, but you need to be able to communicate with others, to the best of your abilities, exactly what is causing your pain. This includes talking with your doctors, your friends, your family, and anyone else who is affected by your pain or who may be able to help with your self-management program.

The biopsychosocial model, by definition, places biological and physical factors right up front. So using this model, we start examining your pain problem by looking at biological and physical factors. Odds are this is the aspect of your pain with which you are most familiar. For most people, it is a biological event that starts the pain problem. You fall at work, hurt your back lifting, twist your ankle, overdo some activity—and then feel pain. Or perhaps you smoke or overeat, and then your breathing is restricted, your joints hurt. These are pain generators: the events, injuries, or conditions that originally set your pain problem in motion. Whatever your pain problem, I'm pretty sure you first noticed it within your physical self. So it only makes sense to start your comprehensive biopsychosocial evaluation of your pain problem with the initial cause. It all starts with the body.

WHY IS IT IMPORTANT TO UNDERSTAND YOUR DIAGNOSIS?

If you know your diagnosis and understand what it means, excellent. But if you find yourself unable to simply describe the physical causes of your pain, this is where we need to start. A wide body of research has shown that if your understanding of your medical problems is vague, you will tend to think the worst about your pain and worry that something is seriously wrong. This in turn launches a series of problematic behaviors. People who believe their pain is a mystery have been shown to have lower self-esteem, sleep more, feel more stress, and be less likely to follow doctors' advice than people who do understand the source of their pain (Williams, Robinson, and Geisser 1994).

Another reason your medical diagnosis is important is that it dictates your treatment. Medical treatment protocols and recommendations follow from the diagnosis, so it is important for you to be familiar with what your doctors believe is generating your pain.

This chapter will help you explore how well you understand the physical causes of your pain. First, I'll guide you in learning more about your diagnosis. We'll explore what others think about the causes of your pain. Finally, you'll evaluate your satisfaction with the care you are receiving and reconsider your role in your medical care.

LEARNING MORE ABOUT YOUR DIAGNOSIS

There are several approaches you can take to learn more about the causes of your pain. Let's start with the person who knows your diagnosis best: your doctor.

Asking Doctors About Your Diagnosis

If you do not know your diagnosis, ask your doctor to tell you in plain English what he believes is causing your pain. Have your doctor put the diagnosis in writing.

Over the years, I have worked with many neurologists, orthopedists, occupational medicine physicians, and pain management specialists, and they have told me that they have reviewed their medical findings and diagnoses with their patients, but still somehow their patients do not know why they are hurting. My experience tells me that some people in pain don't believe what they have been told. They don't see how a muscle, tendon, ligament, or irritated nerve could cause so much pain, so they will say to me that they don't know why they have pain.

Others are so anxious and fearful in the doctor's office that they don't hear what their doctors have said. They listen, but the words don't really sink in.

Another typical complaint is that doctors only spend a few minutes with each patient, and then they are on to the next person. This is a real problem in today's doctors' offices. Be respectful of the position your doctor is in, but also speak up if you have any questions. Write down the key questions you want answered, but keep it to a select few questions.

Getting Your Medical Records

Request a copy of your medical records, and read through them. Most medical records (certainly the initial consultation records) include a section called "Diagnostic Impressions" or "Diagnosis." This is where you find your diagnosis.

Even if you already know and understand your diagnosis, requesting your records is a simple, active step you can take in your pain self-management program. A complete file includes records of all doctor visits and notes, physical therapy notes, specialists' reports, and consultation records. You may have to pay a copying fee to get these, but keep in mind that these are your records, and you need them. Keep a copy of all records, and never give originals away.

Researching Your Diagnosis

Educated and informed people with chronic pain are in a better position to take care of themselves, which is the whole point of this book. Finding information and community resources is one of the tasks that is critical to effectively managing your pain. The Internet is a good place to start, but it's important to stick with reputable Web sites. See Resources at the end of this book for a list of excellent sites that offer research-supported information about various pain conditions and treatments.

EXERCISE 5.1: YOUR DIAGNOSIS

Do you know your diagnosis? In the space below, write down, to the best of your ability, what it is that is physically causing your pain problem.

Compare what you have written with what you have heard your doctor say is the cause of your pain. Are they similar? If they are not, are you concerned that something has been missed? Are you worried that you have a catastrophic medical problem, like a tumor? If so, you need to talk to your physician and express your concerns. Sometimes simple reassurance is all you need. Sometimes it is worthwhile for your doctor to hear your concerns.

LEARNING HOW OTHERS UNDERSTAND YOUR DIAGNOSIS

Pain is not strictly an individual experience, but rather one that involves other people. By understanding how others see your pain—especially what they think is causing it—you begin to manage their experience of your pain. When you manage their experience, you manage your own, because your pain is not yours alone. It affects those around you, which in turn affects you. Being surrounded by friends and family who have a firm grasp on why you are in pain can contribute to a more comfortable and happy environment for all of you. But first you need to determine what your loved ones actually know about your condition. Use the following exercise to ask your spouse, partner, or family what they think is the cause of your pain. You can do this exercise with more than one person.

EXERCISE 5.2: FIND OUT WHAT OTHERS THINK CAUSES YOUR PAIN

Ask your spouse or partner, other family member, or a friend who knows you well to write down in the space below what they believe is the reason you have chronic pain.

Be warned that you might be surprised by what they say or don't say. Try not to be confrontational or judging. Just listen. If they have no response or say they don't know, then it is a wonderful time to share what you know about your diagnosis.

This exercise can be illuminating, reaffirming, or possibly disturbing, but it is always informative. The bottom line is that a lack of understanding and knowledge on the part of your family and friends regarding your pain problem is an additional problem for you. Talk about the results of this exercise. Let your family and friends know what your diagnosis truly is. Explain how you feel about that diagnosis, and discuss how they feel as well. If possible, make sure you are all in agreement as to what causes your pain.

Having a firm handle on your diagnosis and the cause of your pain is an important starting point in your self-management approach to pain rehabilitation. Chapter 12, All in the Family, will look at the impact your pain has had on significant others in your life.

TAKING AN ACTIVE ROLE IN YOUR MEDICAL CARE

Learning more about your diagnosis is just the first step in taking a more active role in your medical evaluation and treatment. This section will help you evaluate what further steps you might need to take.

Take this quick survey now. It will help you determine if you are satisfied with your medical treatment or if you need to spend more time talking with your doctors about your care.

EXERCISE 5.3: LACK OF MEDICAL COMPREHENSIVENESS SCALE

Rate how strongly you agree or disagree with each statement.

My doctors have left no stone unturned in their attempts to treat my pain.

strongly disagree   strongly agree

0   1   2   (3)   4   5   6   7

The medical treatments I have received for my pain have been thorough and comprehensive.

strongly disagree   strongly agree

0   1   (2)   3   4   5   6   7

I have received every reasonable diagnostic test to help determine the cause of my pain (for example, CAT scan, X-rays, myelogram).

strongly disagree   strongly agree

0   1   (2)   3   4   5   6   7

My doctors have tried everything possible to treat my pain problem.

strongly disagree   strongly agree

0   1   (2)   3   4   5   6   7

To score this survey, add up all the numbers you circled. Remember, this is a reverse scored scale. Subtract the total from 28, then divide the result by 4. This is your *lack* of medical comprehensiveness score. This number should be between 0 and 7. Add it to your Pain Scorecard, and we can begin looking at your areas of concern and your personal pain management strengths.

Interpreting Your Score

The higher your score, the more strongly you believe that you have not been thoroughly and comprehensively treated for your chronic pain problem. The lower the score, the more strongly you believe you have had a thorough medical workup.

Level three: 4.2 or more. If you scored 4.2 or higher, you believe you have not been adequately evaluated and feel you have not had the treatment you need to deal with your chronic pain problem. On the Pain Scorecard, a score of 4.2 or greater places you in the level three category, indicating that this is a major area of concern in your overall pain self-management program. If you scored in this category, consider talking with your physician. Ask the questions you need to in order to thoroughly understand your diagnosis and the causes of your pain. Your doctor may ask you what you think needs to be done in order to diagnose and treat your pain problem. Be prepared to answer this question. Try to be as specific as you can. For example, you may believe you need a diagnostic test such as an MRI, or perhaps you are afraid you have the same problem as your uncle who has cancer.

Level two: 2.4 to 4.1.   A score between 2.4 and 4.1 indicates some concern with the adequacy of your medical treatment. On the Pain Scorecard, you would be at level two, indicating you likely have questions about what has been done to treat your pain problem and what needs to be done. In this case, you may choose to make an appointment with your physician to ask questions, or you may do some research on your own to be sure you understand your diagnosis.

Level one: 2.3 or less.   If you scored 2.3 or less, you are at level one, suggesting you believe the diagnosis, treatment, and care for your pain problem has been thorough and comprehensive. This is a major asset and strength in your pain self-management program.

Taking the Next Step

If you scored in level two or three, there are some steps you should take. Ask yourself:

- What is my medical diagnosis?

- What is the usual course of treatment for someone with my diagnosis?

- Are there any treatments that should be done that I have not been offered and that I think would help?

- What diagnostic testing is usually performed in cases like mine? When was the last time I had a diagnostic test done?

- Do I need to see other doctors or specialists?

- Does surgery typically help people with my injury or condition? Has anyone suggested surgery for me?

Next, take these questions and your answers back to your physician and review them together. If you do not feel comfortable discussing these issues with your doctor, read the section on assertive communication in chapter 11.

■ Marie

Marie was a forty-three-year-old married woman with a chronic low back pain problem that had been bothering her for three years. She had seen several physicians but continued to have excruciating pain. On the Lack of Medical Comprehensiveness Scale, she scored a 6.0. She was very concerned because she had not been prescribed physical therapy for more than two years. Marie worried that she was out of shape, having gained forty pounds due to inactivity.

I suggested that Marie write down some important questions to ask her physician at her next appointment. She brought the questions and her Lack of Medical Comprehensiveness survey to her doctor, and together they agreed that Marie would start a physical reconditioning program along with some dietary changes. Marie began to regain some control of her life and felt empowered by the experience.

Marie knew she was worried about having gone so long without physical therapy, but she hadn't been comfortable addressing this fact directly with her doctor. Her high score on the Lack of Medical Comprehensiveness Scale let her know that her concern was legitimate and needed to be addressed. Seeing her score gave her the justification she needed to be more assertive with her doctor. And as it turned out, Marie's doctor was receptive to her concerns, which made it easier for Marie to raise questions in the future.

Overcoming the Patient Dependency Mind-Set

Inadvertently, the medical community has fostered an attitude of dependency on the part of pain patients. Even the word "patient" implies being a passive recipient. A person with this mind-set looks to a doctor for a solution, cure, or fix—which may never come. Many visits to doctors' offices are simply due to a lack of information about pain. Learning which conditions require medical assistance and which you can treat yourself is an important part of the pain self-management approach.

If you are thinking, *I am not a doctor, so I don't know what I need*, remember that this chapter has emphasized the importance of taking an active role in your medical care and asserting yourself to ask the important questions, listen to what is said, and pursue more information if necessary. What you don't know can hurt you. What you don't know, you can find out—whether from your doctor or from other sources. Passivity will not help you feel better.

TO SUM UP

You have now finished part 1 of *The Chronic Pain Care Workbook*. You should have a firm understanding of the basics of chronic pain—what it is, what affects it, and your role in managing it. Now it is time to move on to the specifics of how to improve your experience of chronic pain.

Part 2 will offer exercises to help you identify your strengths and weaknesses in handling your pain. It will help you see where you are currently doing a good job with your pain and where you might do better. It offers information on biological, psychological, and social elements affecting pain and helps you measure the effect of each element on your personal pain experience.

Chapter 6 will explore how and why pain affects energy and fatigue. One of the most common ways to measure quality of life is by how much you can do. How much you can do is determined by your energy levels.

BEHAVIORAL
ASSESSMENT OF PAIN

Your body. Your mind. Your life.

Biological. Psychological. Social.

The hat trick of pain. The three prongs to the salad fork of hurting. The three legs of suffering's bar stool. The triumvirate. The triad. Triangulation. Triathlon. Triage. Three: it's the magic number.

I cannot emphasize this enough: There are three components to your pain. And in order to manage your pain, you must understand all three parts. The road to that understanding is paved with questions. Part 2 of *The Chronic Pain Care Workbook* is that road. In it, you will develop a unique understanding of all aspects of your pain. The scale and survey questions in each chapter make up the components of the Behavioral Assessment of Pain (BAP) questionnaire.

The development of the Behavioral Assessment of Pain questionnaire was my dissertation for my Ph.D. in clinical psychology in 1990, and it has evolved into this book. The BAP questionnaire has been used by pain management professionals throughout the world. Now it's yours.

Benjamin Franklin once said, "That which hurts, also instructs." It is with this in mind that we now move to measuring and assessing your unique pain experience with a critical eye on what it is that you need to learn. Each chapter in part 2 will help you to understand a particular piece of your pain puzzle. Each will include an overview of the topic and then present select questions about your personal pain experiences. You will score your answers and compare them to the responses of more than a thousand other people dealing with chronic pain. Your responses and scores will help you determine what key areas you are struggling with, but they will also help you see where your strengths lie.

Knowledge of your particular struggles and strengths will guide you to the specific treatment options or alternatives that will be most effective for you. Knowledge and insight enable you to feel more in control and help decrease the anxiety of uncertainty. A lack of knowledge and understanding leads to lassitude and inaction—both of which contribute to a feeling of powerlessness. This book is an attempt to empower you. The pain experience is as unique as a fingerprint. By the time you finish reading this book, you should have your fingerprints all over it.

As you go through the exercises, take an extra few seconds to record your results on the Pain Scorecard. This will give you an overview of where to concentrate your energy, and it will mark your progress. Finally, the Pain Scorecard can serve as a guide if you seek professional treatment assistance from a clinician.

CHAPTER 6

Fatigue and Energy Levels

Chronic pain is an energy waster, and it increases your fatigue. Pain makes you tired, and then being tired reduces your tolerance of pain, creating a vicious cycle. That's why energy management is crucial to people in chronic pain.

You spend so much of your energy fighting the pain, worrying about the pain, and trying to live with the pain that you don't have a lot of energy left over. You have no energy to waste. Fatigue is a major enemy to all who are fighting this battle.

Energy provides power to move, and movement promotes well-being and offers a means of responding adaptively to stress and pain. Energy shortages and fatigue lead to a sense of powerlessness that becomes self-defeating. The goal of this chapter is to help you become more aware of your energy resources and help you manage your energy in ways that will empower you. Identifying personal energy wasters is an important component of your pain self-management program, because that knowledge allows you to focus your energy on things that will make you feel better.

MANAGING YOUR ENERGY LEVELS

You didn't always feel the way you do now. And looking back, you may long for those better days. You're not alone in that longing. Here are common comments among people with chronic pain:

I used to be able to work all day, make breakfast, and take care of the chores, and now it is hard to just make my bed in the morning.

I could go all day and not even stop, and by the end of the day I slept like a baby. Then I got up and did it all over again.

I never even thought about what I had the energy to get done. Back then I was always running out of time to do things, not energy.

Frequently, people with chronic pain are challenged in every aspect of day-to-day life, including analyzing how they did things before having pain and comparing that to how they do those same things with pain. But too often, thoughts center on what can't be done, rather than on how to do things differently to accomplish more.

The Way You Do the Things You Do

Fatigue presents a major dilemma for people in chronic pain. From an energy management perspective, the way you do things can be as important as what and how much you actually do. If you don't plan before engaging in some physical activity, you may waste valuable energy—energy that would have been better used in managing your pain. When your energy is limited, it is easy to get sucked into doing more when you feel better (overdoing) and doing less when you feel worse (underdoing). For example, you might wake up on Sunday feeling more energetic than usual and spend the entire afternoon doing yard work. By the end of the day, you are in considerable pain, and you aren't able to do anything around the house for the remainder of the week. By the next weekend, there is a lot of housework to be done, and it's tempting to overdo it again to catch up. The pattern of overdoing/underdoing is very common for people in pain.

The overdoing/underdoing pattern often includes the "damn the torpedoes" outlook, where you think, *I know I am going to hurt anyway, so why not just go for it?* I frequently hear people say, "To hell with the pain. I want to get something done for a change, even if the pain ends up killing me later. I don't care." The problem here is twofold. First, this attitude shows a failure to accept the real fact of having chronic pain. Second, it guarantees a pain flare-up.

Using Relaxation to Renew Energy

Rather than pushing your activity level to the very limit of your energy and driving yourself to exhaustion and a pain flare-up, you can learn to use downtime and relaxation to increase energy. By decreasing stress and learning to relax, you will have more energy to do the things you want to do throughout the day.

Pain influences your level of tension and stress. As pain becomes chronic, it also becomes a constant irritant that can cause permanently elevated levels of muscle tension. Frequently, people tell me that as they begin to anticipate increases in pain, they tense up ahead of time in an effort to cope better. This creates fatigue, and the negative feedback cycle begins: pain leads to tension, which leads to fatigue and then more pain. This cycle depletes your energy resources.

Relaxation is a skill that you need to develop to cope with chronic pain. It helps reduce muscle tension and stress. Learning to relax at will, both quickly and deeply, can improve your pain.

When you're developing any new skill, the more you practice, the better you get. You didn't drive a car expertly the first time you got behind the wheel. But when it comes to relaxing, people tend to think it's simple, so they don't give it a thought. They think they should just be able to do it.

Some people tell me that relaxation does not work for them. When I probe deeper, we discover several problems. For some people, the relaxation method wasn't suited to their needs (for example, they were using deep breathing when they suffered from a respiratory problem). Others tried using the relaxation technique too late in their pain flare-up. (Relaxation helps most when you use it just as the increase in pain becomes noticeable.) Still others did not give the technique enough time and didn't practice it enough to really judge its effectiveness.

Relaxation can take many forms. The most common include breathing, progressive muscle relaxation, guided imagery, and visualization. But there are other methods as well: music, art, reading, yoga, meditation, and exercise. You will see all of these mentioned throughout this book.

There are many different ways to relax your body and quiet your mind, and they won't all work for you the first time you try them. Take those relaxation methods that feel right and work for you, and use them. Let go of the rest.

Using Your Breath

Breathing is an essential part of life. It can help you achieve calmness, reduce tension, and regain energy. Breathing not only brings oxygen into your body but also gets carbon dioxide, a waste product, out of your body. This section will introduce three exercises to help you improve your breathing and your ability to relax.

EXERCISE 6.1: BELLY BREATHING

Learning to breathe from your belly will do you a world of good. Take a minute to try it.

1. Start by getting into a comfortable position lying on your back.

2. Place one hand on your chest and place a book (not a huge one) on your belly.

3. Now breathe. Notice which rises and falls, your hand or the book. If you are a belly breather, the book will be rising and falling. If you are a chest breather, the hand on your chest will be rising and falling. The goal is to be a belly breather. So keep trying until you can make the book rise and fall, even if it takes some effort. Direct your attention to what it feels like to breathe this way.

4. Inhale to the count of five and exhale gently to the count of ten, breathing in and out slowly, deeply, evenly. Repeat four times for an average of four breaths per minute.

5. Stop and relax for a minute if you find yourself getting light-headed or dizzy.

Visual images can help you enhance your belly breathing. Here are a few you can try:

■ When you exhale, imagine a spoonful of your favorite soup is right in front of your mouth. How would you blow on that hot soup to cool it down? Slow and steady. Use this image to regulate the speed of your exhale.

■ Imagine an ocean wave coming onto the beach and then receding back to the ocean. As you inhale, imagine a single wave coming up the sandy beach. As you exhale, imagine that same wave gently going back into the ocean. Repeat this process and notice any change.

■ Try to imagine releasing your body tension as you exhale. Imagine the tension as sand that is slowly slipping out of your body, or see it as a balloon getting smaller as it releases its pressure.

Once you are comfortable with belly breathing, introduce it into your daily life. You can do it anywhere, any time—you don't have to be lying down.

EXERCISE 6.2: BLUE DOTS

Start with some blue dots. These are not special blue dots, just the kind of stickers anyone can get at any office supply store. Put the dots in places where you can see them easily, like on the dashboard of your car, on your fridge, on your bathroom mirror, even on your watch. Place them anywhere you might feel stress or anxiety. Every time you see a blue dot, consider it a reminder to practice your slow belly breathing, or any other relaxation method you find useful.

EXERCISE 6.3: THE SIGH FACTOR

Try sighing right now. What would that look like? Go ahead; no one is looking. If you lifted your shoulders and dropped them while letting out a lungful of air, that would be pretty accurate. People suffering from chronic pain need to sigh more. It's that simple.

People with chronic pain often feel their body has failed them, betrayed them, or become the enemy. In fact, your body hasn't betrayed you; it's just trying to get your attention. Sighing is the body's subconscious way of saying, "Hey, wake up, you're holding me too tight."

Pay attention to sighing—when, where, and why you do it, and under what circumstances—and practice sighing on purpose.

■ Sandy

Sandy was sixty-seven-years old and had suffered a twelve-year battle with chronic fatigue, myofascial pain, and peripheral neuropathy. She was remarkably stoic about her pain and apparently had gotten used to it. However, she looked tense and nervous, and I suspected she was adding to her pain by bracing herself and clenching her teeth. To get a better measure of her pain, I used biofeedback equipment to determine how physically tense her muscles were.

Sandy's muscle tension levels were off the chart, and when I showed her, she was amazed because she felt normal. Over twelve years, she had gotten accustomed to higher and higher levels of tension. Like the proverbial frog in the pot of water over the fire, Sandy knew the water was warm, but she hadn't noticed it was boiling.

She was living with more pain than she needed to. Learning relaxation techniques and using the biofeedback machine to verify her progress, Sandy worked on reducing her pain from the size of a beach ball to the size of a volleyball. After several biofeedback sessions, coupled with deep breathing and muscle reeducation, Sandy's awareness of her body drastically increased. She started to notice how she held her head, how she sat. She could see the muscle tension levels change with practice. When she sighed, the biofeedback scores plummeted, and she lit up like a little kid.

It may take a lifetime to learn how to do things inefficiently, but it doesn't take a lifetime to undo those lessons. After one session with the biofeedback machine, Sandy was asking when she could come back and do it again. After so many years of being more and more tense and thinking that it was normal, Sandy was relearning the basics.

My hope is that this book will serve as your feedback mechanism, so you can see where you are and what you need to do to function better and live a quality life. The Pain Scorecard is your gauge, your thermometer. You can see where you are in relation to others. You can see how you change over time. You can see where you are having trouble. And you can see where you are doing well. It allows you to direct your limited energy into things that can most benefit you.

EXERCISE AND CHRONIC PAIN

One of the most useful places you can focus your energy is exercise. Many people with chronic pain are physically inactive—a tragic irony, because inactivity is a more dangerous enemy than pain.

Pain teaches many people to rest and reduce their activities. It seems only natural. But natural or not, excessive rest is not good for anyone. Excessive rest—not using your muscles—will cause not only a loss of muscle strength, but also a loss of flexibility and endurance. The way to combat such deficits is through mild exercise.

We have learned from many studies in the field of physiotherapy that when you move less, you begin to lose strength in your muscles. We call this *deconditioning*. The more you rest, the more your muscles weaken. As time goes on, any activity becomes difficult and causes additional pain. As Helen Hayes, a famous Broadway theater star, once said, "The more you rest, the more you rust."

A negative feedback cycle can develop as pain leads to inactivity and inactivity leads to more pain. Ironically, the new pain you experience can be from inactivity and not necessarily from the original pain generator. This is an important point because many people lump all pain into one category: *the* pain that they have lived with for so long. They fail to appreciate that the soreness that comes from increased activity after being sedentary is not their original pain, nor is it coming from their primary pain generator. This new pain is likely perfectly normal and related to deconditioning rather than to the pain problem. If you lump all your pain together, you make your pain problem bigger than it has to be. By separating pain generators into categories (the pain of a herniated disk or nerve problem, for example, versus the new pain of a sore muscle or twisted ankle), you can gain some perspective and potential control.

Acute pain tells you to take it easy and rest. However, in most cases, if you employ this strategy even when pain lasts longer than a week, you begin to break down physically. With minimal to no movement, your body reduces its output of *endorphins* and *serotonin* (the body's natural painkillers), which in turn reduces your ability to produce *GABA* (a neurotransmitter that inhibits pain). You start to lose your ability to regulate your own experience of pain.

Many people with pain have tried some form of exercise in the past but stopped because of increased pain levels. Frequently, they have been told to exercise until it hurts and then stop. The message often is "no pain, no gain." With this approach comes the idea that hurt means harm, and unfortunately, this notion is reinforced by some health care providers unfamiliar with working with people with chronic pain conditions.

You will feel discomfort starting any new activity or exercise. But don't mistake normal soreness for harm. Soreness and discomfort does not mean you have harmed yourself. It is just a sign that you are doing something that your body is not used to. Muscle soreness is known to peak one to two days after increased exercise. It is important to anticipate and plan for this so that you don't interpret it as a worsening of your chronic pain. Muscle soreness can occasionally aggravate your fears about reinjury. (We'll discuss these fears further in chapter 8.) Remember that fluctuations in pain are expected in response to exercise.

Some people, by their very natures, try to do too much too soon. These people push themselves too hard, often feeling good at the time but then feeling much worse for days after. A more effective approach is to gradually and steadily work up to therapeutic levels of activity.

For all these reasons, a mild exercise program is an important intervention strategy for overcoming both physical deconditioning and the belief that any activity beyond the minimal is physically damaging. Of course, you must talk with your physician to ensure exercise is not contraindicated.

There has been a lot of research looking at the benefits of exercise for those who live with chronic pain. The overall conclusions suggest that exercise and physical activity are much more important than you may have thought in managing your pain. Regular exercise can be a very effective weapon in coping with chronic pain. Plus, it's just plain good for you.

Getting Started and Staying Motivated

It's natural to be worried about hurting yourself or making your pain worse. But with input from your doctor and physical therapist, you can safely exercise with the knowledge that your pain isn't serving a useful protective purpose. Remember that regular exercise actually eases chronic pain for many people.

Consult your doctor and physical therapist for help designing an exercise program that meets your specific needs. Your doctor will likely recommend various stretching, strengthening, and aerobic exercises. Swimming, biking, and walking are often good choices. Exercises that help you relax—such as meditation and yoga—may be helpful, too.

However, getting started is not enough. Even if you recognize the benefits of exercise, staying motivated can be a challenge. Stay focused. Remember to start slowly and gradually increase over time. Don't rush into a strenuous workout before your body is ready. Pace yourself and be consistent. The intensity of the workout is less important than the fact that you do it regularly, especially if you have severe pain.

There are a few tricks you can use to keep yourself motivated. Build your exercise program around activities that you enjoy. If you enjoy mellow group energy, try a yoga class. If you like a fast pace and pop music, try aerobics or even a spin class. If you hate being indoors, try walking instead of using a treadmill in a gym. If you hate complicated machines, get some good shoes for walking and a simple set of weights for home.

Exercising with a buddy can also be helpful as a motivator and as a distraction. Find a friend, neighbor, or colleague who wants to get in better shape and work out together, encouraging each other and making exercise more fun. And remember that walking around the block is exercise. As your energy increases and your mood improves, exercise may truly become fun.

Benefits of Regular, Moderate Exercise

A gradual increase in movement and exercise can alter your attitudes about pain and improve your quality of life. As tough as it may be to start an exercise program, your body will thank you. Find out what to expect, then get moving. Consider what exercise has been shown to do for people with chronic pain:

Improve flexibility, strength, and endurance.   These benefits apply not only to exercising but also to performing life's activities. There is a large body of evidence confirming that this goal can be accomplished for a majority of patients with chronic pain. You are less likely to be plagued with aches and pains if you have a full range of motion.

Reduce the intensity of pain.   Studies of exercise have found that pain intensity decreases between 10 percent and 50 percent in people who maintain an exercise program (Hayden et al. 2005). Exercise can reduce discomfort.

Reduce fears and concerns associated with movement in general.   Once you learn to distinguish between your true chronic pain and the normal discomfort that comes from increased activity, you will likely discover that gentle exercise does not contribute to your chronic pain and in fact helps relieve it. This, in turn, can help you feel freer and less fearful about being more active in general, opening up a whole new world for you.

Stimulate the release of endorphins.   Exercise seems to stimulate the body's natural defense against pain through endorphins, natural pain-relieving substances. Endorphins slow pain signals to the brain and can also help with mood problems such as anxiety and depression—conditions that can make chronic pain more difficult to control.

Improve function.   Exercise is a tool to improve your ability to function, and it can boost your energy level. Regular exercise can actually give you more energy to cope with chronic pain. Weight reduction is a by-product of exercise, and maintaining a healthy weight is a major pain management strategy. Exercise burns calories, which can help you drop excess pounds. Remember that ten pounds of weight puts one hundred pounds of pressure on the spine. Exercise also helps improve or maintain musculoskeletal and cardiovascular function and build strength. The stronger your muscles, the more force and load you'll take off your bones, tendons, ligaments, and cartilage, and the more relief you'll feel.

Improve emotional life.   Exercise can help you feel better emotionally, by providing a sense of productivity and satisfaction. Exercise can also improve the quality of your sleep. Regular exercise can lower your stress hormones, resulting in better sleep. Blood and oxygen flow to your muscles improves with exercise and contributes to an overall sense of well-being. Looking and feeling better helps your confidence and can improve your self-image. Setting exercise goals and meeting them can give a sense of accomplishment previously lost for many people in pain.

Stretching for Better Flexibility

Your exercise routine should include stretching exercises to improve flexibility and restore normal range of motion. A good method is *static stretching*. It requires only minimal training and can be done without a therapist. You must hold static stretches for at least thirty seconds in order to achieve changes in flexibility, and you can get additional benefit by repeating these exercises in up to four sets. Three sessions of stretching per week will improve your flexibility, but you can make even greater gains in flexibility by stretching five times per week. After you have increased your flexibility through a training program, one session of stretching per week is enough to maintain the increases.

Here are a few basic stretches from which most anybody can benefit:

Calf stretch.   Placing your hands on a wall, extend one leg behind you gently while maintaining your heel flat on the floor. Hold this for fifteen to thirty seconds. Then switch sides.

Calf raise.   Standing on the edge of a stair or step, gently let your weight push you down, then raise up on your toes. Repeat this five to eight times.

Shoulder roll.   In an upright position, lift your shoulders up and down, keeping your shoulders back. Do this five to ten times.

Neck rotation.   Put your left hand on your right shoulder to prevent a twisting motion. Turn your head away from your hand, holding this position for fifteen to thirty seconds. Switch sides and repeat.

You can get more information on stretching from books, Web sites, and of course your physical therapist.

Targeting Cardiovascular Endurance

Improving endurance is a reasonable exercise goal for people with pain. You can increase your cardiovascular endurance by exercising for a prolonged period of time at a less-than-all-out level. Types of exercise that improve aerobic condition include walking, running, dancing, cycling, swimming, and using endurance training equipment such as treadmills, exercise bikes, or stair machines. To improve your endurance, aim to exercise three times per week for at least fifteen minutes at 60 percent to 75 percent of the maximum heart rate for your age (see table 6.1).

The High Price of Inactivity

If the benefits of exercise and physical movement are not motivating enough, here are some reasons inactivity is dangerous.

In an article published by the *Western Journal of Medicine* in 1984, Walter M. Bortz II pointed out the extensive problems caused by what he called "the disuse syndrome," or deconditioning. Bortz's work was backed up by Paul J. Corcoran in 1991 (also in the *Western Journal of Medicine*). Of course, the importance here is that chronic pain teaches you to be inactive (a state Bortz called disuse). But what does that inactivity do?

Inactivity:

■   Reduces muscle fiber

■   Reduces oxygen intake

■   Raises blood pressure

■   Decreases the normal range of motion in joints

■   Contributes to osteoporosis

■   Fuels anxiety, depression, and anger

■   Decreases lung capacity

Bortz concluded that inactivity plays a pervasive role in lack of wellness.

One of the most extraordinary aspects of the human body is its resilience. Its ability to recoup its losses is enormous. There is still time to turn your life around. Start a program of movement, exercise, and physical activity today.

Table 6.1: Target Heart Rate by Age

Age	Age-Adjusted Maximum Heart Rate	60%	75%
20	190	114	143
21	189	113	142
22	188	113	141
23	187	112	140
24	186	112	140
25	185	111	139
26	184	110	138
27	183	110	137
28	182	109	137
29	181	109	136
30	180	108	135
31	179	107	134
32	178	107	134
33	177	106	133
34	176	106	132
35	175	105	131
36	174	104	131
37	173	104	130
38	172	103	129
39	171	103	128
40	170	102	128
41	169	101	127
42	168	101	126
43	167	100	125
44	166	100	125
45	165	99	124
46	164	98	123
47	163	98	122
48	162	97	122
49	161	97	121
50	160	96	120
51	159	95	119
52	158	95	119
53	157	94	118
54	156	94	117
55	155	93	116
56	154	92	116
57	153	92	115
58	152	91	114
59	151	91	113
60	150	90	113
61	149	89	112
62	148	89	111
63	147	88	110
64	146	88	110
65	144	86	108
66	143	86	107
67	142	85	107
68	141	85	106
69	140	84	105
70	139	83	104

Choosing an Exercise Program

Your exercise program needs to be achievable, beneficial, and safe. To launch your exercise program, choose an activity that suits your individual needs.

Walking is an excellent activity for just about anyone. In winter, you can use a treadmill or walk in indoor shopping centers. In summer, you can walk outside, ideally on a flat surface such as a school track, a flat road, or an interesting area of your town. You may want to couple walking with music (iPods and MP3 players are great for this). Use a timer if time, rather than distance, is your measure of exercise. This will help you pace yourself and resist pushing on too far and too hard. Walking in a warm pool is another option. Your area may have clinics that have these warm walking pools. Check with your local YMCA or hospital, or ask your physician for a referral. If you are overweight or really hate the thought of exercising, this is a good start.

Gentle stretching and strengthening exercises are a good choice for people with chronic pain. Yoga can be of value to almost everyone. Pilates, an exercise program that emphasizes strengthening the core muscles that support the torso and back, is another good option. You can also try a structured program like that offered by gyms such as Curves. The important thing is that you get started.

■ Jerry

Jerry was a cowboy. Yes, there really are working cowboys in this world, especially in Nevada. He was the true essence of the Marlboro man, minus the smoking. But Jerry had a classic back injury from years of riding horses and working on the ranch. He was diagnosed with degenerative disk disease.

Jerry had been a very active man all of his life. A true cowboy, he would get up at 4:30 every morning to get the campfire started and the coffee brewing. All day, he would be on his horse, working the Nevada high desert to find cows that had been put out to graze. The years of riding in the saddle had taken their toll.

When Jerry's pain got so bad that he could no longer sit in the saddle and work, he came to me for help. When I suggested that he needed to get some exercise, he laughed and said, "I never exercised before, so why do I need to now?"

Jerry had gotten most of his movement and exercise from working as a cowboy. But he had been incapacitated for the past eight months and was doing virtually nothing but lying in bed. When I mentioned exercise, I explained I wasn't asking him to run a marathon or lift weights for the Olympics. I wanted him to ease into a routine of movement that was appropriate for his age, ability, and pain level.

I asked Jerry to start slowly and get into a warm pool and simply start walking in the water. He thought I was crazy but signed up for it. On the third day of the pool walking, he came to me and said that he was feeling a little bit better. Within weeks, he gradually moved to a land-based walking program and said he was feeling much better.

Jerry had figured that working on a ranch meant he never needed to exercise. That was a reasonable thought when he was working, but it had carried over to his nonworking life, where it was not so reasonable. Today, Jerry still has his pain, but he continues to walk because it makes him feel good.

Pain and Activity Level

Your level of activity and the level of pain you experience is related, but how? The elevator/escalator metaphor is a useful way to think about this relationship. If you're an elevator person, you push yourself hard, and your pain level shoots up along with your activity level. Then, when you can't take it anymore, the elevator plummets: your activity level drops off abruptly, and your pain level follows.

You don't want to get on the elevator. Take the escalator instead. Increase your activity level gradually. You may move more slowly, but at least you will get where you want to go. When an elevator is strained too far, it plummets back to the bottom. When an escalator gets overloaded, it simply stops wherever it is, and you continue to your destination on your own, or you simply step off. You do not go hurtling to the bottom.

Activity pacing is your escalator. It is an important way to break the negative feedback cycle of overactivity, pain flare-ups, and underactivity.

EXERCISE 6.4: GRAPH YOUR PAIN AND ACTIVITY LEVELS

Let's see if you are an elevator person or an escalator person. Use this graph to track your activity level against your pain level over the course of two weeks. For activity level, 0 would represent no activity and 10 would represent strenuous activity. For pain intensity, use the 0 to 10 scale you learned in chapter 4.

GRAPHING PAIN AND OVERALL DAILY ACTIVITY LEVELS

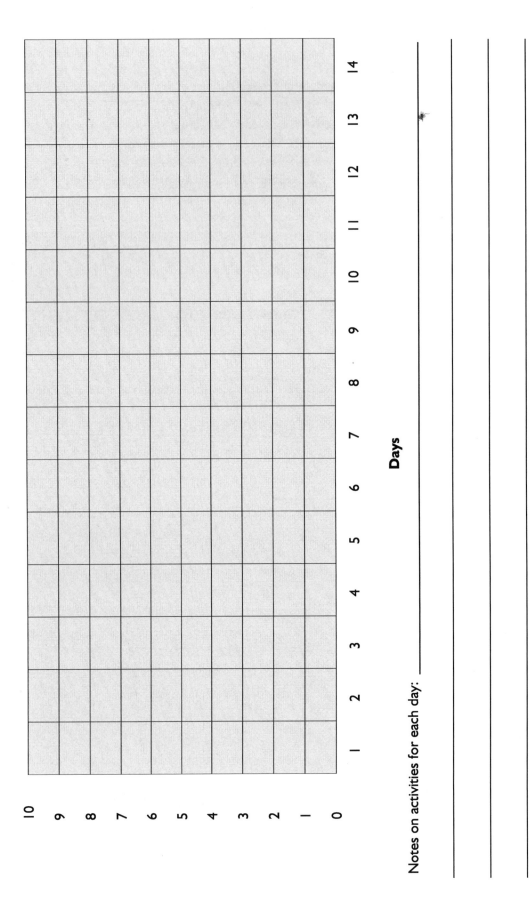

Days

Notes on activities for each day:

Compare your worksheet to figures 6.1 and 6.2. If your graph looks like figure 6.1, you are on a dangerous elevator ride. If your graph looks more like figure 6.2, you are on a gentler, more reliable escalator.

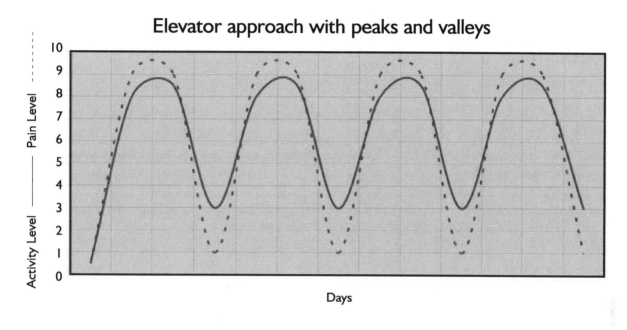

Figure 6.1: Elevator Approach (Peaks and Valleys)

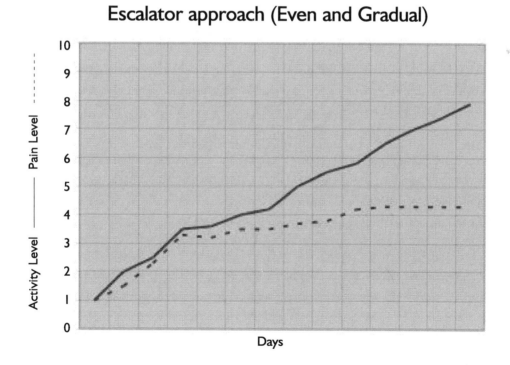

Figure 6.2: Escalator Approach (Even and Gradual)

Activity monitoring helps you become more aware of the types of activities you are doing and how your activity level relates to your pain level. This data will be important if you want to maintain the same activity level you had before you developed chronic pain. You want to make sure that you do not put yourself at risk for further injury and pain by setting your goals too high. Conversely, setting your goals too low means you run the risk of getting little to no benefit from the exercise you do take on.

Riding the Elevator: Peaks and Valleys of Pain and Activity

Most of the people who come through my practice are elevator people. They suffer the extreme highs and lows of what they consider activity-induced pain levels. But while they may share the basic pattern, they don't always share the same reasons for the pattern—or the same level of motivation to solve the problem.

Different people get on the elevator for different reasons. Here are just a few:

- Feeling guilty that other people have to perform tasks

- Having a tough time accepting that they can't do everything

- Thinking in rigid or black-and-white terms

- Catastrophic thinking

■ Greg

Greg was fifty-seven-years old and raising his three young grandchildren. Ever since a slip and fall at work a few years back, he had been fighting chronic low back pain. Greg was a typical person in pain in that he paired activity and pain—he was an elevator person. The more he did, the more he hurt. But he was unusual in that the paired association of activity and pain came not from any of the reasons above. Instead, Greg had a problem with procrastination.

Procrastination was nothing new for Greg. It had plagued him his entire life, not just since the pain problem began. In school, he would put off studying, then cram all night just before a test. Chores around his house built up until they turned into full-out repairs. Bills went unpaid until threatening final notices arrived. But procrastination worked for him. He got good grades in school, he managed to get friends to help him with repairs on his house, and the power never got turned off.

Suddenly Greg had to contend with a pain problem. He continued to put things off. But time keeps moving. He procrastinated until he hit a wall, and he could no longer put off all the things he had been neglecting. As is typical for elevator people, Greg ended up getting everything done by overdoing it—but he had to, because he had procrastinated. He soldiered through the pain and got done what he needed to get done. He hopped on the elevator, which took him to high levels of activity in a very short time, and the net result was a crash down to the basement. He was on the couch for several days recovering.

Procrastination is Greg's nature. It's familiar. It's his comfort mode. He had never looked at procrastination as a problem he was responsible for perpetuating, and he had never considered the link between procrastination and pain. It had never occurred to him that if he used pacing and just did a little every day, he wouldn't have the crash.

Once he discovered pacing, he discovered a whole new world. Now Greg stays on top of things. He's working from home, his house doesn't need repairs, the power company isn't wasting paper reminding him to pay his bills—and he is living more comfortably.

Riding the Escalator: Slowly Increasing Activity

Successfully riding the escalator of pain control relies on the concept of activity pacing. Pacing means increasing your activity level gradually so that you build a tolerance for more activity. It also means taking a break before you need it and not letting your pain get out of control. Here are some suggestions on how to use the escalator metaphor to improve your health and well-being by breaking the association between "the more I do" and "the more I hurt."

First, select a physical activity that is realistic, achievable, and enjoyable to you (for example, swimming, walking, or bicycling). Then establish a baseline or tolerance level for this activity. To do this, perform the activity until pain, weakness, or fatigue prevents you from continuing. Then stop—don't overdo it. The level at which you stopped is your baseline or tolerance level. You can measure the level in terms of time or distance, whichever makes sense for that activity (for example, number of minutes you walked). Take these baseline readings for about three days to get an average reading for this activity.

Now establish an activity level starting point for your escalator. Take your average baseline level and cut that in half. Use this as your starting point. For example, if your baseline tolerance level for walking is twenty minutes, your starting point would be ten minutes of walking. To maximize your chances of success (at least initially), start low and then build up. Don't be frustrated by starting low; you will be increasing these levels over time.

Next, set your goal. What would you like to be able to do? Your target will help determine how steep the escalator will be. Increase your activity levels often and in small steps, rather than occasionally and in large steps. If the escalator starts looking like an elevator, either your goal is set too high or you are moving upward too quickly. You may need to revise your goal and adjust your escalator to be more realistic.

If your goal is realistic and your escalator is not too steep, you can use the escalator (rather than your pain) as your guide. Try not to use pain as an excuse to avoid movement. Increase your activity levels according to the escalator model and not how you are feeling on any given day. Remember to pat yourself on the back for each step and especially when you accomplish your goal. Resist the temptation to discount the positive and say that it was nothing.

Kim

Kim was a twenty-nine-year-old single woman who was diagnosed with piriformis syndrome, a condition where pain is felt in the distribution of the sciatic nerve, radiating from the buttocks down to the back of the thigh, but there is no back pain. Kim used to run every day for stress relief, but pain had turned her sedentary. She hated the extra weight she was carrying and the way she got out of breath with the simplest tasks. But it wasn't as if she could just start running again. She'd tried that and ended up in the hospital. A physical therapist had worked with her on stretching the piriformis muscle, and this helped. But her core problem was that after the last hospital stay, she was convinced that the more she did, the more she would hurt.

I worked with Kim on a reasonable plan of activity pacing. Since she liked to walk and jog, we started with taking a baseline reading for walking around a track. She walked until pain stopped her and she felt weak. She did this for three days, averaging about two laps. We concluded that walking one lap, or half of her baseline, was about right as a starting point. On day one, she was to walk one lap around a track at the local high school. On day two, she was to do the same. On day three, she was to walk one and a half laps. On day four, she was to do the same. Her goal was to reach one mile (four laps) a day. I asked her to graph her activity each day so she could see her progress.

The problem was that Kim missed being active. She was impatient. She walked her one lap around the track on day one. She thought that this was nothing like her old self, and got frustrated. On day three, she decided to really push it, and she walked four laps around the track. She jumped off the escalator and onto the elevator, and then spent the next two days in bed recovering. Does this sound familiar?

Kim went back to her peaks and valleys. The next time she came in, I worked with her to find a pacing schedule that allowed a little flexibility. If she felt good after meeting the day's goal, she could do a little more, but not much. I added dashed lines a little above and a little below her daily target on her chart. This gave her a little more control and flexibility and allowed her to choose a comfortable pace. She could do a little more than the target on any given day or a little less, depending on how she felt. But it made sure she did something each day without doing too much. She had to stay within the dashed lines of the graph. Figure 6.3 shows Kim's revised chart.

As she followed the new chart, Kim noticed her pain did not increase significantly. It pretty much stayed the same day to day. Her pain was manageable, and she did not need to increase her medications. She also noticed she was not as irritable or cranky as she had been before she started exercising. Her mood was good. Over time, she did more, but she didn't hurt more. The paired association of "the more I do" and "the more I hurt" had been broken, and Kim was active again—and without increases in her pain like she was used to having. She was able to maintain her target level of activity and no longer had the peaks-and-valleys pain experience. She found that even when she had a flare-up, it was not as bad as it had been before.

Not Going Up at All: Low Activity

Kim is an example of someone who had been riding an elevator and switched to an escalator. She was motivated to regain the physical fitness she had enjoyed before her chronic pain developed—she just needed help pacing herself so she could achieve that goal. But I also have worked with people whose normal activity levels before pain were simply low. These are the sedentary types who wouldn't likely bother with either an escalator or an elevator because they don't particularly care to go up.

These low-energy people don't have a problem with peaks and valleys. But to improve their pain condition, the prescription is the same: the escalator. Movement is life. People who aren't physically active and moving risk depression, obesity and the related strain on the joints, diabetes, high blood pressure, and heart problems—none of which is going to improve their pain any. The irony is that inactivity doesn't always mean less pain; sometimes, it means more pain. If you are one of these people, you need to slowly increase your level of physical activity beyond the old levels. A sedentary lifestyle may have seemed to work before pain, but now rest is certainly not best.

Kim's Activity Pacing Chart with Flexibility

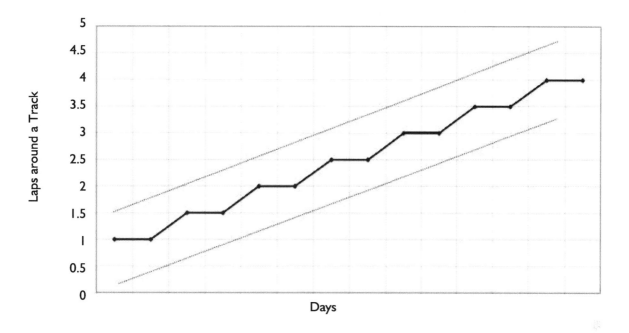

Figure 6.3: Kim's Activity Pacing Chart with Flexibility

Comparing Activity Levels Before and During Pain

Whether an increase in pain is due to extreme fluctuations in activity level or an overall activity level that is too low, the important measurement is the difference between your activity levels before pain and since the pain became chronic. There are people who had high activity levels before pain and people who had low activity levels before pain. The people with high activity levels before pain often suffer more, because the difference between their old selves and new selves is greater. People who had low activity levels before pain often find they get in a rut with the pain. They are used to not moving, and they find it difficult to get out of the rut of being sedentary.

Some people will try to maintain the same schedules they kept before the pain started. They often end up exhausted and need excessive time to rest and regain energy. In many cases, it even makes the pain worse. Ironically, it is often the people who try to maintain their old schedules who most feel that others do not understand them. Despite their efforts to appear as they were, they feel others are not sensitive to their plight. "Nobody really knows how bad this pain is," they say, and yet they believe that if they acted in accordance with the way they really feel, nobody would want to be around them. These people waste energy in wishing for care, and, at the same time, use more energy to guard against alienating friends and family.

Evaluating the Impact of Pain on Your Productivity

When you start an exercise program, you're not exercising just for the sake of exercise. You get all the health benefits I mentioned earlier in the chapter. Your mood and self-esteem improve. But most important, you extend your *productivity*, or your capacity to do whatever it is you choose to do in your life. You become more productive at work, at home, and in the things you do just for fun.

This exercise will help you identify whether you have a fatigue and energy management problem as the result of poor activity pacing. I want to explore with you what you are most concerned about when your pain flares up.

EXERCISE 6.5: REDUCED PRODUCTIVITY SCALE

When your pain increases sharply, how concerned are you that
your pain will interfere with other activities

not at all concerned						very concerned	
0	1	2	3	4	5	6	7

you will not accomplish anything else the rest of the day

not at all concerned						very concerned	
0	1	2	3	4	5	6	7

the rest of the day will be shot

not at all concerned						very concerned	
0	1	2	3	4	5	6	7

you will not get anything done

not at all concerned						very concerned	
0	1	2	3	4	5	6	7

To score this survey, add up all the numbers you circled, then divide the result by 4. This is your reduced productivity score. This number should be between 0 and 7. Add your score to your Pain Scorecard.

Interpreting Your Score

Level three: 4.9 or more.   A high score on the Reduced Productivity Scale suggests you are vulnerable to poor activity pacing and often overdo it. You probably tend to push through pain and keep going too long in one activity. You run the risk of developing a peak-and-valley pattern of pain and activity. Failing to plan before engaging in physical activities or going about things in an uncoordinated way—trying to do a variety of tasks at the same time—increases your vulnerability to pain flare-ups. Many people with chronic pain force themselves to complete a task because that is the way they have always done things, and they got away with it in the past.

Following this pattern of activity, you may begin to think, *The more I do, the more I hurt*, and the corollary, *The less I do, the less I hurt*. These thought patterns and activity patterns are further reinforced when your pain levels increase and decrease based on your activity levels.

A high score on this scale, reflecting a fear of decreased productivity, is shown through my research to be highly correlated with increased levels of depression (see chapter 11) and catastrophizing about your pain (see chapter 8). In essence, inappropriate activity patterns set you up for feeling out of control and lead to emotional suffering. A variety of vicious cycles emerge when even one thing goes wrong.

At this level, poor activity planning and lack of pacing become a major form of energy depletion, raising your fatigue level. Fatigue in turn decreases your ability to cope with pain, leading to frustration and depression.

Level two: 2.7 to 4.8. If you scored at this level on the Reduced Productivity Scale, you are like most people who have chronic pain. The peak-and-valley activity pattern is still likely to be an issue but perhaps not as significant. It may be something you do, but it is not an ingrained pattern.

Although peaks and valleys are not such a problem for you as they are for somebody who scores at level three, pacing can still be a considerable challenge for you. Many people deplete their energy reserves by procrastinating—putting off today what you can do tomorrow. But when tomorrow comes, you usually don't feel any better. And now you have to do whatever it is you were putting off.

Avoidance behavior is perhaps the defining characteristic of procrastinators. You think, *I know I am going to hurt if I do all the laundry today, so I'll do it tomorrow.* See Janine's story below; procrastination is the trap she fell into. She tried to postpone the seemingly inevitable adverse consequences until another day. But she found that by pacing activities more appropriately and spreading them out over time, she could avoid the big push later. That way, she also avoided the big flare-up.

Imagine that you have only so much energy for a given day's journey, just as you have a limited amount of gas in your car's tank. Use it wisely. Running out of gas means you stop moving. Efficiency is the key. Worrying and anticipating future pain flare-ups is comparable to racing around town, revving up your engine and wasting a lot of gas—and getting nowhere.

You may be thinking, *I'll just rest and take it easy.* But excessive inactivity or immobility does not necessarily fill up your tank and give you more energy. Like so many things in life, helpful rest is a matter of degree. Extensive rest is not best.

Of course, resting and taking a break as a means of activity pacing is productive and helpful. And rest following activity is a nice reward, but lying in bed for hours or days on end is an energy waster. The key is to pace yourself and work efficiently so you don't run out of gas.

Level one: 2.6 or less. Scores of 2.6 or less suggest minimal risk for poor pacing and problems with over-doing activities. A level one score is a major asset and strength in your overall pain self-management program.

▧ *Robin*

Robin was a marathon runner who had gone through back surgery followed by foot problems. Before surgery, she had been a very active woman who won marathon races at the age of forty-five. She was commonly described as "high-energy" and relished the description.

Robin had invested a lot of her identity in being active; it was a major part of how she saw herself. Then, suddenly, she was faced with change. She needed to let go of her old self and her old achievements and come to terms with where she was in the present. But coming to terms with such change and accepting a new identity are difficult issues. Robin needed to adapt and be flexible.

Being adaptable means not simply doing things the way you always did but instead adapting to the changing environment, using new facts and information to set and reach goals. Inflexibility and rigid thinking get in the way when the evidence shows new limitations are a reality.

Letting go of the old self is hard. But it does not have to mean quitting and giving up. Robin struggled with depression and grieved over the loss of the person she had been. Over time, she moved toward accepting her condition and focusing on modifying her life with chronic pain. Today, she works with several local charities setting up marathon races as fund-raisers. While she no longer runs in these races, she is still part of the event and the action.

■ Janine

Janine is a typical example of a person with a pacing problem. She had major neck and shoulder pain that traveled down to her left arm and hand. She was diagnosed with a cervical strain and thoracic outlet syndrome after being rear-ended in a car accident. When she came to me for help, she had been struggling with pain for the past eleven months. Her husband was a long-haul truck driver and was only home on the weekends. Janine always looked forward to seeing him. They had been married only a few years.

Janine was something of a perfectionist. Her home was always clean. I joked that I probably could eat off her floor, and she quickly quipped, "Of course you could."

Prior to her pain, Janine had always been able to do whatever she wanted for as long as she wanted, with no negative consequences worse than mild soreness. With her neck and shoulder pain, however, she was unable to keep the house as clean as she liked it, and this bothered her greatly—to the point that she became mildly depressed.

Talking with Janine, I noticed she had started to develop a pattern in her weekly routine. Her pain stopped her from cleaning excessively every day (not a bad thing), but she found that by the end of the week her house was "intolerable" and "filthy." Her pain had taught her that the more she did, the more she hurt, so she put off the housework until the day before her husband would come home. But she wanted him to see that the pain hadn't changed who she was, so the morning before his return, she would take several pain pills and push hard all day to get the house in order. She would end up exhausted and in tremendous pain by the time her husband arrived.

Janine would be in bed all weekend with the major pain flare-up that followed her excessive activity, and she missed spending time with her husband. Her husband was frustrated, and their relationship worsened. In our sessions, Janine and I discussed how poor planning set her up for a major pain flare-up and subsequent disappointment and depression.

In time, Janine began to pace herself better. She planned chores in smaller steps and set realistic priorities for herself. She ended up having more energy on the weekends, when her husband was home.

SLEEP, ENERGY, AND CHRONIC PAIN

Poor sleep and interruptions in sleep can drastically decrease your energy levels and your ability to function. Sleep interference and anxiety over not getting a restful night's sleep are huge problems for people in pain. People who can't sleep have a lot of valid complaints, but most fall into two categories: inability to initiate or maintain sleep at night (*insomnia*), and inability to maintain wakefulness during the day (excessive daytime sleepiness). People who have chronic pain often have both complaints, but one of these usually predominates.

Most people who don't struggle with pain seldom even think about sleep. Bedtime comes, and they lie down, go to sleep, and wake up hours later rested and refreshed. But for people who do struggle with pain, sleep is an ongoing challenge of sometimes epic proportions. To make matters worse, treating the pain does not always fix the sleep problem. While the two are related, they must be treated separately.

Sleep is an essential dimension of human health. And good sleep routines often play a major role in effective pain management. Therefore, of course, developing good sleep routines is a major pain self-management strategy.

Before we go further in the discussion of sleep, let's see if sleep is a problem for you. Take this sleep quiz before you read on.

EXERCISE 6.6: SLEEP INTERFERENCE SCALE

Sleep Onset

■ Do you have trouble falling asleep?   yes   no

■ Does it take you more than ten to fifteen minutes to fall asleep?   yes   no

■ Do you go to bed at different times each night?   yes   no

The more yes responses, the more likely you have a sleep onset problem.

Sleep Maintenance

■ Do you have interruptions in your sleep?   yes   no

■ Do you have trouble staying asleep?   yes   no

■ Do you wake up earlier than normal and have difficulty falling back to sleep?   yes   no

■ Do you have nightmares that wake you from sleep?   yes   no

The more yes responses, the more likely you have a sleep maintenance problem.

Sleep Duration

■ Has the number of hours you typically sleep (decreased or increased)   yes   no
significantly over time?

■ Do you wake up feeling tired and not rested?   yes   no

Interpreting Your Score

Yes responses suggest sleep is not serving a restorative function, and poor sleep may be a key factor in the maintenance and worsening of your chronic pain problem. If you answered yes to zero, one, or two items, score yourself in level one on the Pain Scorecard. If you answered yes to three or four items, score yourself in level two. If you responded with yes to five or more items, place your score in level three.

Chronic Pain and Poor Sleep Patterns

One obvious problem for people in pain is just getting comfortable enough to fall asleep. People with chronic back and neck pain seem to be the most at risk for developing sleep problems, since they have difficulty finding comfortable sleeping positions. They toss and turn, because they can't stay in one position for very long without their pain levels increasing.

The most common complaint of people with chronic pain is that pain wakes them up. And this complaint has been backed up by research showing that people with chronic pain have more nighttime awakenings than pain-free people (Currie et al. 2000). You probably knew that already. People with chronic pain are primarily awakened by the pain, but they are also easily awakened by external factors like noise or a lumpy bed. They are constantly having to fall asleep over and over every night.

There are many ways chronic pain contributes to sleep problems. The most common include the injury itself, nighttime pain, medications, decreased daytime activity, inconsistency in schedules and routines, weight gain, and problems with mood and anxiety.

Pain at night is not the only contributor to sleep problems. Lack of sleep cuts two ways. Increased daytime pain can cause a night of poor sleep or be caused by a night of poor sleep. Pain on either or both ends of sleep affects pain, which affects sleep, and so on.

Sleep and Behavior

Though sleep disturbances tend to begin because of pain, they have a tendency to create behavior habits that go far beyond the pain in perpetuating the problem. In other words, it may be your pain that starts your problem, but your actions keep it going. Common factors that contribute to sleep disturbances regardless of pain include a variable sleep schedule, a preoccupation with sleep, daytime napping, and inaccurate beliefs developed in response to poor sleep.

Sleep and Mood

While we know that anxiety can keep us awake at night, most of us think of depression as causing people to sleep more. But it can have the opposite effect, especially for people in pain. Major depression can cause anyone to sleep less. Depression plus chronic pain is a recipe for insomnia.

People suffering with chronic pain are at risk of self-perpetuating cycles of sleep disruption, increased pain, and depression. Poor sleep can lead to a decrease in activities (physical and social), leading to a decrease in the amount of social support and an increase in depression. People with chronic pain often experience significant mood disturbance along with sleep disturbance. Psychological distress (depression, anger, or anxiety) is often worse for people in pain who can't sleep than it is for those who can.

Sleep Efficiency

In his excellent book on improving sleep, *Insomnia: Psychological Assessment and Management* (1993), Charles Morin recommends you determine your "sleep efficiency ratio," or the percentage of your time in bed you spend actually sleeping. To calculate your sleep efficiency ratio for a given night, divide your total sleep time by the total amount of time you spent in bed and multiply the result by one hundred. Generally, as your sleep improves, your sleep efficiency ratio will increase. The average sleep ratio for good sleepers is between 85 and 95 percent. A person with an average sleep efficiency ratio below 80 percent is a poor sleeper.

Keeping a Sleep Journal

Self-awareness is the beginning of self-management. The first step in treating any sleep disturbance is to keep a log of sleep. You may think you know how you sleep, but it is human nature to remember the worst the most vividly. Keeping a log will give you a less biased view of your sleep patterns. Make at least twenty-one photocopies of the Sleep Journal worksheet. Fill out the worksheet each day for the next three weeks.

SLEEP JOURNAL

Date: _____

Last night's sleep:

time lights out _____

minutes until sleep _____

time up and out of bed this morning _____

number of sleep interruptions _____

total hours slept _____

total time spent in bed _____

sleep efficiency ratio (hours slept divided by hours spent in bed times 100) _____

how rested upon awakening, on a scale of 0 through 10 _____

sleep medications used?   yes   no

average pain level today, on a scale of 0 through 10 _____

EXERCISE 6.7: SLEEP EFFICIENCY AND PAIN

What is the relationship between your sleep efficiency ratio and your pain level? See the chart on the next page. Once you have kept a sleep journal for three weeks, you can use this graph to chart the relationship visually. For each of the twenty-one days, mark your sleep efficiency ratio, then draw a line connecting the marks. Using a different color pen, do the same for your pain levels. How do the two lines relate?

Getting a Better Night's Sleep

Poor sleep patterns don't need to be permanent. There is a lot you can do to get a better night's sleep almost every night. In this section, I'll share some of the most effective tools for improving your sleep.

Understanding Factors That Affect Sleep

When your sleep is good, you don't think about it. So you may have never learned much about sleep before it became a problem. Here are a few key points you need to understand about sleep.

Substance use.   What you put into your body affects the quality and quantity of your sleep. Caffeine, nicotine, and alcohol all change your sleep patterns. Caffeine and nicotine are stimulants and can keep you awake. Alcohol may help you get to sleep (it is a central nervous system depressant), but it disrupts sleep a few hours later. Modify your use of these substances, and you will sleep better.

Exercise.   What you do with your body also affects the quality and quantity of your sleep. Exercise raises your body temperature and then lowers it over time. Because of this, exercising right before sleep can keep you awake. But exercising four to eight hours before you go to sleep can enhance your sleep greatly. Regular exercise can be a great help in reducing your pain and setting the stage for restorative sleep.

Napping.   When you're tired, you want to sleep. Sleeping at night is fine. But sleeping during the day—napping—can quickly become a habit. The later in the day you nap, the less likely it is that you are going to get a good night's sleep. If you feel you must nap, experiment with the timing and duration of your naps. Some people find that short morning naps help their overall sleep patterns.

Routines.   People with chronic pain often develop elaborate daily routines to cope with the pain. Examples include spending a great deal of time in bed during the day to counteract joint and muscle pain, sleeping in the living room chair at night for the same reason, and getting up during the night or early morning to take pain medications. Needless to say, these routines often run counter to the effective behavioral management of sleep.

SLEEP EFFICIENCY AND PAIN

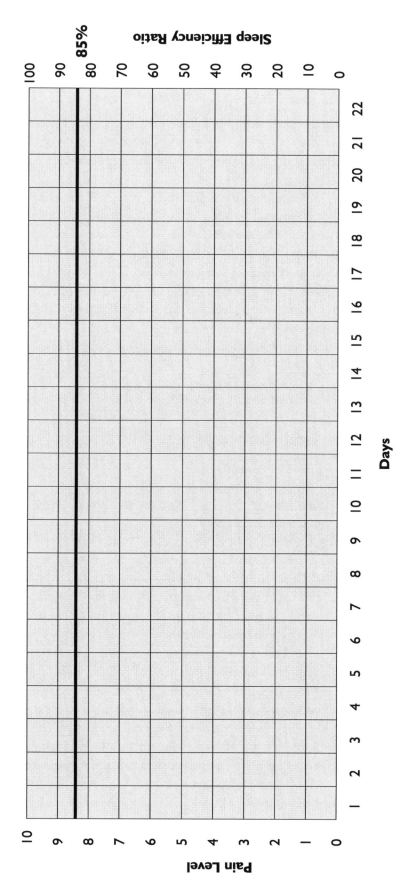

Sleep efficiency goal is 85% or higher.

Restricting Time Spent in Bed

Restriction of time spent in bed seems counterintuitive. What you want is more sleep, not less, right? But limiting the amount of time you spend in bed to the time you spend actually sleeping can be an effective treatment of insomnia.

Your *sleep window* is the portion of your time spent in bed that you actually spend sleeping. Expanding your sleep window helps you concentrate your sleep into shorter periods of time spent in bed. This will make your sleep less fragmented and interrupted. There are two ways you can expand your sleep window: either delay going to bed or get up earlier in the morning. The result of sleep restriction is to create a state of mild sleep deprivation, which speeds the onset of sleep and increases the depth and quality of the sleep attained within the sleep window (Spielman, Saskin, and Thorpy 1987; Currie et al. 2000; Morin 1993).

Over the course of four to five weeks, aim to gradually increase your sleep window until you achieve 85 percent sleep efficiency. Note that in the short term, increasing your sleep window does not necessarily mean getting more sleep. Sleeping three hours out of four spent in bed gives you a sleep efficiency ratio of 75 percent. Sleeping four hours out of eight spent in bed gives you more sleep but a poorer sleep efficiency ratio (50 percent). Your goal is to increase your sleep efficiency ratio to 85 percent. For the time being, don't worry about the number of hours of sleep you're getting. In the long run, better sleep efficiency will lead to more hours of sleep.

Read on for suggestions that will help you expand your sleep window.

Building a Healthy Sleep Routine

Most of us don't go to sleep just because we are tired. We go to bed out of habit or because the eleven o'clock news is over or our partner has gone to bed. But if you are not tired, it is not a good time to try to go to sleep, so remember, go to bed when you are tired.

Similarly, too many of us don't go to bed just to sleep. We read, eat, watch TV, listen to music, or work. This isn't a good idea. Don't use your bed for anything but sleep. Don't even use it to worry. The only exception to this rule is sexual activity. Don't worry, you can still have sex in bed.

But just because you are using your bed for nothing but sleep (and sex), that doesn't mean you lie in bed for hours trying to sleep. If you don't fall asleep within ten to fifteen minutes, get up and do something nonstimulating so you don't fall back on these other activities (especially worrying) in bed. If you wake up at night and can't go back to sleep within ten to fifteen minutes, get up and do something nonstimulating. Read, watch TV, eat—just don't do it in bed.

Whenever possible, keep a consistent routine about when you go to bed and when you get up. Set your alarm and get up at the same time each morning, no matter how much sleep you got during the night and no matter how tired you are. Try to go to sleep at the same time every night, but if you can't sleep, get up. You may not be able to find a consistent bedtime each night in the beginning, but stick to a consistent out-of-bed time anyway. That may be tough, since you will be tired if you didn't get much sleep the night before, but do it anyway with the knowledge that being tired will help you get to sleep the next night and will help you develop healthy sleep routines.

Building routines is the goal. "Routine" means ongoing. It does not mean one good night's sleep. You'll need to stick with it.

Support from others will help you follow the rules for sleeping better. Get the support of your family, if you can. Have them remind you why it is important that you stick to your guns. Have them help you go to bed and get up at appropriate times. Have them help keep you awake when you are tired outside the appropriate times for sleep.

Evaluating Your Sleeping Environment

Where you sleep affects the quality and duration of your sleep. A good pillow, a good mattress, and a dark, quiet room are necessities. Even the best mattress should be replaced after about ten years.

Different kinds of pillows and bedding work for people with different ailments. For example, people with cervical spine disease can be helped by the added support of a cervical or oat-shell pillow. People with neuropathic pain may benefit from "tenting" bedding so that it does not aggravate sore areas.

Make sure your bedroom is as dark and quiet as possible. White-noise machines or recordings of peaceful sounds or music can be helpful for just about anyone, as can extra-dark drapes. Taping aluminum foil to the windows can be an effective and inexpensive way to make your bedroom dark.

Cultivating Relaxation

Relaxation reduces stress. You can't have anxiety and relaxation at the same time; your body won't let you. Take a little time each night before you try to sleep to relax. Breathing, meditating, praying, listening to relaxation tapes: there are many ways to relax.

Working on Thoughts and Ideas About Sleep

There is not a lot in your life that isn't affected by your thoughts, ideas, and beliefs. Sleep is no exception. Over time, it is easy to establish irrational and unrealistic, yet powerful, beliefs and fears when it comes to sleep (or lack of sleep, as the case usually is). People suffering from insomnia tend to focus on the negative consequences of not sleeping. Focusing on the problem without doing anything to change it can make you feel hopeless and out of control.

If you've had ongoing problems falling asleep, you are familiar with the cycle of not sleeping and then worrying about not sleeping and then not sleeping because you're busy worrying. Add pain to this mix of anxiety and sleep disturbance, and you get even more irrational fears and counterproductive ideas. The worry is increased because you aren't just worried about sleeping; you're worried that because you aren't sleeping, you will hurt more.

People in pain also run the risk of blaming daytime problems—such as fatigue or an inability to concentrate—on lack of sleep. These problems may be side effects of medication or may be related to the pain problem, but the person in pain may believe they are caused by lack of sleep. This adds more anxiety and more pressure to fall asleep, which decreases the chances of getting to sleep.

People in pain have heard a lot about resting, and with good reason. Rest is good for healing. But people with insomnia may also believe that they must get eight hours of sleep every night in order to be healthy. They therefore feel that it makes sense to nap or just stay in bed the day after a poor night's sleep. They cancel the day's activities in the name of rest, but they are really just shrinking their world to include nothing but their pain.

People in chronic pain who have insomnia often don't see alternatives. They believe they will never sleep well again so long as they are in pain. In fact, this is not the case—unless they do nothing to change the situation.

Sleep Medication

Changing thoughts and actions is often enough to resolve sleep disturbances. But not always. Medication can be of great help if you have short-term insomnia. However, long-term use of sleep medications, or *hypnotics*, is not a solution for sleep problems caused by chronic pain.

The effects of sleep medications can last for different amounts of time. Some work only for an hour; others work for several hours. The short-acting hypnotics metabolize more quickly, decreasing the odds of hangover, and they help get you to sleep, but they won't help you stay asleep for the full night. The longer-acting hypnotics will help you stay asleep, but the effects can carry over into daytime hours as well, causing problems the next day, and these medications can accumulate in your system over time.

The side effects for different hypnotics must also be taken into account. Some can make you sluggish or cause memory loss. Some increase the risks associated with hypotension (very low blood pressure), restlessness, anxiety, and confusion. Of course, there may be additional risks when hypnotics are combined with other medications. Talk to a doctor before you begin taking any medication.

Don't Give Up

Perhaps you have been struggling with sleep for a long time now, but don't get discouraged. Aggressive treatment of sleep problems is critical. A problem in the past does not have to be a problem in the future. Many factors that contribute to poor sleep can be changed with a little work on your part. Sometimes the best treatment combines a little bit of cognitive work (changing your thoughts and beliefs) and behavioral work (changing your habits and actions). Feel free to mix and match suggestions to suit your needs. Or work with a professional who can tailor a program just for you. Such professionals could include psychologists or doctors who work in sleep labs.

HOW LOSS AND GRIEF AFFECT ENERGY

Energy levels are often diminished when people experience a sense of loss and grief with chronic pain. Pain can dramatically change your life. Through this book, I am trying to help you regain as much of your old self as you can, but the fact remains that because of your chronic pain, you have lost some part of who you used to be.

Grieving is a natural part of life, but prolonged grieving may signal other problems outside the chronic pain experience. These other emotional issues and problems often can be helped through professional intervention. If you find that grieving has been a primary experience for you for some time, I strongly recommend that you seek some professional help. (See my recommendations in Resources about support groups.)

NUTRITION AND ENERGY

Nutrition is a cornerstone of an effective pain management program. Yet it is often overlooked. Fighting pain is hard work for your body, even if that body is doing nothing more than lying on the couch. And in order for your body to have the energy to wage that fight, it needs fuel. The better the fuel, the more efficient the body.

While many people will work with their pain management team to choose medications, fine-tune their dosages, deal with their side effects, and monitor their effectiveness, they balk at doing the same with their food and drink. They believe one form of ingested substance (medication) will change their life, while another (food or drink) won't. I completely understand this way of thinking, but it's worth questioning.

"Tell me what you eat and I'll tell you who you are" (Jean-Anthelme Brillat-Savarin) is an adage that has much truth in pain self-management. Healthy eating is a means of gaining an upper hand on pain flare-ups. Good food choices can reduce your pain and improve the negative side effects of pain (such as fatigue, weight gain, and digestive problems). And on the opposite side of this coin, unhealthy eating (and poor nutrition) will increase pain and suffering.

You may have one of two basic problems: eating too little due to pain or eating too much due to pain. Eating too little can deplete your energy and diminish your strength and endurance. When you eat a poor diet, muscle tissue can break down, and this can contribute to perpetuating pain cycles. Eating too much because you're bored or because you need comfort can also worsen your pain through weight gain.

The field of nutrition is confusing at best, but there are a few basic principles that have not changed over years of research. First, drink plenty of water. The human body is largely made up of water, and flushing the body with fresh water and staying hydrated is a simple way to stay healthy and improve your energy. Drink a full glass of water every two hours. Second, follow the recommendations in the food pyramid developed by the U.S. Department of Agriculture. These include emphasizing whole grains and low-fat sources of protein, eating lots of fruit and vegetables, and reducing your intake of sweets and sugary foods. Fruits and vegetables are an excellent source of vitamins, minerals, and dietary fiber.

Food is fuel. So nutrition is a key factor in energy management. If your body is using all its energy just to fight pain, you won't have energy left over for any other part of your life. You will find yourself sedentary. This can lead to weight gain (or unhealthy weight loss), deconditioning, diabetes, heart disease, and depression—and it won't do a bit of good for your pain.

Movement is life. I work every day with people who want life and therefore choose to move. They learn that everything they put in their body influences the way they live. They avoid dieting and the stress it puts on the body. They drink plenty of water. They exercise without overdoing it. They decrease the pressure on their spine and joints by maintaining a healthy weight through proper nutrition and exercise. (Remember that ten pounds of weight puts one hundred pounds of pressure on the spine.) These are long-term goals that yield long-term improvements.

■ Mike

Mike is a fifty-one-year-old married man who works as a pain specialist. He spent his life eating the typical American diet (meat, potatoes, bread, milk, cheese, and desserts). Since Mike looked fit and never had serious health problems, he saw no reason to change his diet. But he knew better. He knew how diet affects energy. So during the course of writing a workbook on chronic pain, and to support his wife's choice of a healthier life, Mike switched to a raw-food diet.

The switch was a big change for him, and one he thought would be hard to maintain. Except he felt so darn good. If there were a pill that made him feel this good, he would be dependent. His weight is down, his skin looks younger, even his breathing has improved. But the best part is the energy. Changing his diet has made Mike a new man. A side effect for Mike was the discovery that he is allergic to dairy products. He spent decades with swelling and inflammation he had grown to see as normal—until it was gone.

Raw food is not the answer for everyone. But for Mike, looking closely at what fuels him, what he puts into his body, has been a major eye-opener.

MUSCULAR DISCOMFORT AND ENERGY

It's hard to be active when your muscles hurt. And movement may exacerbate muscle pain. But movement is life. Frequently, people suffering from pain have some form of muscular complaint as part of the pain problem. As part of the many negative feedback cycles, muscle tension and fatigue play a major role in exacerbating and making your pain problem worse. This questionnaire will help you determine whether muscular tension contributes to your pain, limits your activities, and diminishes your energy levels. In the section about interpreting your score, I'll provide suggestions about breaking the link between muscular tension and fatigue.

EXERCISE 6.8: MUSCULAR DISCOMFORT SCALE

Over the past two weeks how often have you experienced the following symptoms?

muscle twitching

not at all							very often
0	1	2	3	4	5	6	7

restlessness

not at all							very often
0	1	2	3	4	5	6	7

fatigue

not at all							very often
0	1	2	3	4	5	6	7

muscle tension or tightness

not at all							very often
0	1	2	3	4	5	6	7

sore muscles

not at all							very often
0	1	2	3	4	5	6	7

To score this survey, add up all the numbers you circled, then divide the result by 5. This is your muscular discomfort score. This number should be between 0 and 7. Place this score on the Pain Scorecard.

Interpreting Your Score

Level three: 5 or more. If you scored at this level, you may have significant problems with myofascial and soft tissue pain. People who score high on this scale often have high levels of anxiety and concern about their body. Being tense and restless is taxing on your energy reserves. Chances are you're bracing yourself, making your pain worse. You are living with more tension and tightness than you need. You may be your own worst enemy. Relaxation training and muscle release work may be very effective for you. Physical therapy and massage are often helpful, along with movement exercises such as Pilates and yoga.

Level two: 3.4 to 4.9. If you scored at level two, muscle tension is a significant—although not extreme—problem for you, and the suggestions for people at level three also apply to you.

Level one: 3.3 or less. Scores less than 3.3 suggest minimal muscular discomfort. With low scores, muscle-related problems may not be of significant concern. Look to other pain generators as the source of your pain.

TO SUM UP

As you have learned, energy is affected by a variety of factors: how you do things, pacing, relaxation, breathing, activity and exercise levels, sleep, mood, thoughts, and, of course, pain. All these factors influence energy, and energy and fatigue play a major role in your pain experience.

This chapter gave you a lot of information about each of these factors in hopes of showing you elements in your life that can be improved. Perhaps your pain can't be cured. But maybe your pain can be improved with less tension, better pacing, mild exercise, healthier sleep patterns, and more realistic expectations. Knowing how each factor influences pain and understanding what you are doing well and what you might improve, you can change your experience of pain for the better.

In chapter 7, we move away from energy and into the subject of medication. Medication also affects energy, but it does much more. Every person with whom I have worked has turned to pain medication at one time or another. Most had questions about using such substances. Many had trouble with what they were taking. Chapter 7 covers the questions and concerns I see most in my practice.

CHAPTER 7

Medication

Ideally, you could take a pill and feel better. And sometimes that is just how it works. But not always. Not by a long shot. Medication alone does not resolve the total chronic pain experience. Although medication can be a valuable component of a pain management plan, it is best used as part of a multidisciplinary treatment program that addresses the biopsychosocial components of your total pain experience. Remember, the ultimate goal of treatment is to help you function and improve the quality of your life.

If you have chronic pain, you probably already know something about medications. But let's start with a basic overview and work from there.

MEDICATIONS USED TO TREAT CHRONIC PAIN

For most people, the first line of defense against a pain flare-up is medication. Medications for chronic pain fall into several categories. Each category of medications has a unique use—and characteristic risks and side effects.

Nonnarcotic Analgesics

Nonnarcotic analgesics include aspirin, acetaminophen (Tylenol), and nonsteroidal anti-inflammatory drugs (NSAIDs) such as ibuprofen (Advil, Motrin). They are most effective for inflammatory pain, such as rheumatoid arthritis and osteoarthritis. They can be helpful with musculoskeletal pain, myofascial pain, and headaches. The long-term use of these medications can present problems in some people in the form of stomach and intestinal distress.

Antidepressants

Antidepressants—including Zoloft (sertraline), Prozac (fluoxetine), Desyrel (trazodone), Sinequan (doxepin), and Tofranil (imipramine)—can be surprisingly effective in relieving pain in some people, possibly due to their effect on neurotransmitters such as serotonin and norepinephrine. Some antidepressants, including amitriptyline (Elavil), have been used to treat headaches and neuropathic pain.

One positive side effect of certain types of antidepressants is sedation, which can assist people in pain who also have trouble sleeping. If you use antidepressants, be aware that they usually take from ten days to a month before they have any effect.

Anticonvulsants

Anticonvulsant medications—for example, gabapentin (Neurontin), topiramate (Topamax), and oxcarbazepine (Trileptal)—have been used to treat various pain conditions, such as migraine headaches, trigeminal neuralgia, diabetic neuropathy, and chronic pain of a neurogenic (nerve) origin.

Muscle Relaxants

Muscle relaxants—for example, cyclobenzaprine (Flexeril) and methocarbamol (Robaxin)—are used to treat muscle spasms and can be useful in the early treatment of acute muscle-related pain. Long-term use of these medications may not be appropriate due to negative side effects, including addiction and withdrawal effects.

Antianxiety Medications

Antianxiety and sedative medications—for example, diazepam (Valium), clonazepam (Klonopin), and lorazepam (Ativan)—provide short-term benefits to people in acute pain by decreasing muscle spasms and reducing anxiety related to treatment procedures. Long-term use of these medications for chronic pain may be problematic and should be discussed with a physician.

Opioids

Opioids mimic the actions of natural chemicals the body produces to relieve pain. Opioids fall into two categories, short acting and longer acting.

Short-acting opioids include morphine sulfate (Roxanol), codeine, hydrocodone (Vicodin, Lortab, Norco, Vicoprofen, and Zydone), oxycodone (Roxicodone, OxyIR, Percocet, Tylox, and Percodan), hydromorphone (Dilaudid), oxymorphone (Numorphan), and fentanyl (Actiq).

Pharmacologically long-acting opioids are those that last longer due to an inherent property of the drug. These include methadone (Dolophine, Methadose) and levorphanol (Levo-Dromoran). *Pharmaceutically long-acting* opioids are formulated by the manufacturer or pharmacist to be released slowly.

These include sustained-release morphine (Oramorph SR, MS Contin, Kadian, and AVINZA), sustained-release oxycodone (OxyContin), and transdermal fentanyl (Duragesic patch).

There are a variety of ways to get medication into your system. It may be taken orally, injected, applied topically and absorbed through the skin, taken rectally (as suppositories), or inhaled.

Any medication can cause side effects, many of which are unpleasant. These can include constipation, dizziness, and impaired concentration. You must weigh the benefits of the medication against the side effects. It is important to let your doctors know if you have any problems taking your medicine so that they can find ways to help manage the side effects.

A CLOSER LOOK AT OPIOIDS

The most common class of pain medications is opioids, and opioids come with some problems. But you can avoid these problems by educating yourself.

Even with the best medical and psychological techniques, some patients with chronic pain may need opioid medication. The strategy for using medications for pain management is usually to progress from weaker to stronger, depending on your unique response. Generally, you would start with a nonsteroidal anti-inflammatory drug, then make a gradual transition to a mild opioid medication if the NSAID was not effective in holding back the pain. If you got only minimal pain relief from mild opioids, you would typically shift to stronger opioids.

Why not just start with the big guns? The answer lies in the potential pitfalls of opiates: tolerance, dependence, and addiction.

Tolerance

Different people respond to opioids differently. Your body metabolizes and reacts to the medications based on your unique biology. But the most common reaction to opioids is tolerance. *Tolerance* is simply your body getting used to a medication. Over time, when you use a medication regularly, the effect of the drug wanes, and you end up needing higher doses to achieve the same effect. Similarly, the side effects of the drug—nausea, constipation, sedation, and unclear thinking, with opioids—become less noticeable over time when the drug is taken regularly (not so with intermittent, "as-needed" dosing). This is why so many people can take opioids regularly and still function normally.

Dependence

Dependence is just what it sounds like: over time, when you use a drug consistently, you can grow dependent on it. Dependence may be physical, where your body adapts to the chemical and you experience withdrawal if you reduce your dosage or stop taking it altogether, or the dependence may be psychological. Psychological dependence is an emotional state that may occur as you become accustomed to taking a drug to experience its positive effects. You may believe you need the drug even if your body never becomes physically dependent on it.

Addiction

Addiction occurs when changes in the neurochemicals in the brain cause a compulsion to get and take the drugs that overrides any consequences of which the user might be aware. Addiction is an ongoing problem that has a tendency to come back over and over. It is chronic with a high potential for relapse.

Addiction is a major fear for pain patients, but it is not as common as most people think. Addiction is especially rare in people who take their medication as recommended. Physical dependency and tolerance are much more likely outcomes, even for those with addiction in their personal or family histories. Monitoring from a doctor is essential for people with such histories, however. Proper use of pain medications reduces the likelihood of addiction.

It is only natural for you to experience tolerance, dependence, or even withdrawal with opioids. (Indeed, you may experience all three even with nonaddictive, nonopioid, nonprescription drugs.) None of these spell addiction in and of themselves. Addiction comes paired with compulsion. No compulsion, no addiction.

Addiction arises from a not-entirely-understood set of circumstances. Genetics, or family history, plays a role. So does gender; males are more prone to addiction than females. Ignorance is also a factor. If you don't know how to take your medications properly and others don't point out that you aren't taking them properly, it is easy to take them incorrectly—intentionally or unintentionally. Chemistry also matters: the addictiveness of the chemicals, the delivery form, and the time of release have an effect. Combinations also have a role; not all drugs play well together.

Not all drugs are equally addictive. In general, a drug such as cocaine is more addictive than opioids, which are more addictive than alcohol. Intravenous use is more addictive than oral. And short-acting, rapid-onset medications are more addictive than slow-onset, long-acting ones.

Pseudoaddiction

Pseudoaddiction is also a risk with opioid use. With *pseudoaddiction*, a person's behavior can look like addiction, but it may actually be an attempt at better pain control. A pseudoaddict takes an extra pill or rations pills for flare-ups in reaction to or in anticipation of pain, not for a better high.

EXERCISE 7.1: OPIOID RISK TOOL

Are you at risk for developing problems with prescription opioid medications? This questionnaire, developed by Lynn Webster and Rebecca Webster (2005), will help you answer that question.

Mark each box that applies.

		Female	Male
Family history of substance abuse			
alcohol	☐	1	3
illegal drugs	☐	2	3
prescription drugs	☐	4	4
Personal history of substance abuse			
alcohol	☐	3	3
illegal drugs	☐	4	4
prescription drugs	☐	5	5
Age (mark box if sixteen to forty-five)	☐	1	1
History of preadolescent sexual abuse	☐	3	0
Psychological disease			
attention deficit disorder, obsessive-compulsive disorder, bipolar disorder, schizophrenia	☐	2	2
depression	☐	1	1

Total score: _____4_____

For each box that you checked, give yourself the number of points listed under your gender. Then add up your total score. A score of 0 to 3 suggests low risk, 4 to 7 suggests moderate risk, and a range of 8 to 26 suggests high risk.

GETTING EFFECTIVE PAIN RELIEF FROM MEDICATION

How you take your medications is as important as what medications you take. Have you ever wondered why some medications say "Take one every four hours" and others say "Take as needed"? This is an important distinction when pain becomes chronic. Chances are, you are like most people who have pain: you take your pain pills only when you can no longer stand the pain. Perhaps you think, *If I take my medications every four hours, I will be using more than if I just take them when I need them, and I definitely don't want to become addicted.* So you push through the initial pain warning signs and wait until you reach your pain tolerance limit—that point when you can no longer stand it. Many people think that if they tough it out, it won't be as bad next time. That doesn't work. In fact, the opposite is true. Pain weakens a person. It weakens the immune system, and it does not build character.

Many people find that they take their pills and they get some relief. That pattern and medication schedule continues over days and weeks. What they learn is that taking a pill reduces their pain and a reduction in pain is the direct result of taking medication. Through this experience, you can develop what I call the "peaks and valleys" problem with pain medications. Pain levels increase to an intolerable level and then decrease rapidly when you take a short-acting pain medication such as Vicodin. The blood levels of the short-acting narcotic pain medications also follow this pattern, in that they peak in the bloodstream within four hours after use and then drop precipitously after four hours, requiring a repeat dose of the medication.

Avoiding Medication Peaks and Valleys

Taking one short-acting pain pill at a time can give tremendous relief when you first start taking the pills, but over time, as you develop a tolerance, you need to take two or three pills to get the same effect. Before you know it, you are taking more pills by the day's end than you would have if you had taken one every four hours. Pain reduction gradually decreases over time, so taking pills only reduces pain from a 7 to, say, a 5 instead of a 1 on the 0 to 10 point scale.

Taking pain medications only on an as-needed basis—the *pain-contingent* approach—essentially creates a powerful set of beliefs and expectations that, over time, can reinforce taking more medications and increase suffering. By taking pain medications only when pain is severe, you undergo a conditioning process in which the behavior of taking medication is reinforced by the relief that follows taking medication. The pitfall is that your pain management is less effective and you run an increased risk of tolerance and dependence.

An alternative, supported by Wilbert Fordyce (1976), a pioneering researcher in chronic pain management at the University of Washington, is a *time-contingent* approach. With this approach, you take medications on a regular schedule, like once in the morning and once in the evening, rather than only when you really hurt. This offers the dual advantages of maintaining more consistent blood levels of medication and also reducing the pain level peaks and valleys of the pain-contingent approach (see figure 7.1).

Pain relieving effects of short-acting versus time released medications

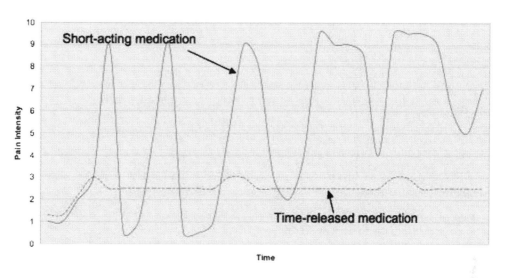

Figure 7.1: Pain Relieving Effects of Short-Acting Versus Time-Contingent Medications

PREVENTING ADDICTION: YOUR BEST DEFENSE

When you take the medications as directed by a physician, addiction to opioids used to treat chronic pain is rare. But even so, it's much better to prevent addiction than to have to treat it later. A proactive approach will help you stay on the path of proper pain medication use.

Tell your doctor about current and past problems you've had with pain medications. If you've ever misused alcohol, recreational drugs, or other prescription medications, be sure to mention those experiences, too.

Take your medications exactly as your doctor prescribed them. Your doctor will tell you about doses and schedules when giving you the prescription. If you're not sure how to take a medication, ask your doctor or pharmacist. If you don't understand the instructions, ask your doctor to repeat the answer using different words. Don't leave the office until you're certain you know how to take your medication.

Talk to your doctor if the pain relief you're getting from medication isn't adequate. You and your doctor can decide what changes to make in your routine.

Ask your doctor about using scheduled doses of long-acting medications rather than taking short-acting medications on an as-needed basis. Sticking to a schedule helps you avoid taking more medication than you can safely handle. Develop a system for taking your medication on schedule and stick to it. Following a routine helps you avoid double doses and other mistakes.

Talk to your doctor about foods, beverages, and other medications to avoid while you take the pain medication. Alcohol, some foods, and some common over-the-counter remedies can alter the effects of the pain medication, so ask about these first.

In his excellent book *The War on Pain* (2000), Dr. Scott Fishman, chief of the Division of Pain Medicine at the University of California at Davis, points out that long-acting opioids are not as likely to give you the euphoric feeling you get with short-acting opioids. The euphoria is what many addicts are compelled to achieve. If you don't have the euphoria, you don't get the addiction.

People with addictions are driven by compulsion. They are preoccupied and distracted, concentrating on getting and using the drug, not on living their lives. This is not a good quality of life. Addiction leads to lower quality of life than pain does.

The long-acting or time-released opioids don't totally get rid of pain, but they do enough good that you can get through the day more easily—without the same risk. You still hurt, but you function. With increased function and no addiction, the quality of your life can be drastically improved.

Now, opioid dependence is a different story. Opioid dependence does not cause the same distraction and compulsion as opioid addiction. In fact, people dependent on opioids, people who have a consistent but controlled intake of medication, may find life dramatically improved. These people often report feeling as if they have reclaimed their life. The pain is there, but muted. They rejoin life—work, friends, family, and activities. Their lives are better. The life of an addict is worse. There is a simple but profound distinction between addiction and dependence.

ESTABLISHING YOUR TRUSTWORTHINESS AND CREDIBILITY

The issue of addiction leads us to the important concepts of trustworthiness and credibility. These are nowhere more important than in the area of pain medications. Because pain is subjective and invisible, your doctors must depend on you to accurately describe your pain and its intensity. Doctors may become suspicious of possible unstated motives for requesting pain medications, including drug seeking, establishing disability status, and avoiding responsibilities. It's in your best interest to present as clear and accurate a picture of your pain experience as you can. Perhaps more than in any other area of medicine, your physicians rely on you having the proper motive in seeking pain management care. You must remember to be accurate in your testimony about your symptoms; don't exaggerate. Show that you will be responsible and follow through with your doctor's recommendations. Sharing the worksheets in this book with your doctor can help demonstrate your commitment to a comprehensive pain management plan.

HELPING YOUR DOCTOR HELP YOU: MAKING A CONTRACT

Your physician wants success in your pain management. She needs to know if things are not working and enjoys hearing when they are working well. For this reason, when it comes to medications, it is your job to keep your physician informed as to your progress (or lack thereof).

Upon graduating medical school, doctors take an oath to help their patients. They swear to do—to the best of their abilities—what they think will most improve their patients' lives. Doctors also know about addiction and its sometimes deadly effects. They don't want to make your life worse. They walk a tightrope between pain control and addiction when they prescribe addictive substances. You can help them balance on that tightrope by helping them help you. After all, you don't want to become a drug addict any more than they want to enable you to do so.

Similarly, you don't want to come across as an addict (especially if you aren't). There are red flags physicians look for that you might raise without meaning to. Communication is key.

Let your doctor know that you understand the risks and real rewards of prescription pain medication. The following contract may be useful for you and your physician if you think you are a candidate for opioid medications to manage your pain. It may save your physician time and help you establish credibility and avoid the trap of being seen and treated as an addict.

SAMPLE MEDICATION CONTRACT

I understand that medications (opioids or narcotics) can assist in pain management. I am wondering if these medications could be part of my pain self-management and rehabilitation plan, but I need your help to make sure I am a good candidate for medications.

I have the following pain management goals, and I hope that medications can assist me in reaching these goals:

- I want to increase my ability to function in meaningful activities of my life, such as being part of family activities, having social experiences, and engaging in play and hobbies again.

- I want to improve my mood and quality of life by once again doing things that used to be fun, by feeling happier, and by feeling more a part of life again.

- I want to improve my ability to engage in work (paid or unpaid).

I am aware of the following:

- Complete pain relief and elimination is rarely achieved. I know that research has shown that narcotics reduce pain by about 30 percent in about 50 percent of those people taking them. This will roughly translate into a change of about two or three points on a pain intensity scale of 0 to 10, assuming I am in the moderate to severe pain range.

- Medications are only one treatment in a multifaceted approach to treating my pain.

- If I am a candidate for opioid analgesics, I should have regular follow-up visits with you.

I agree that I will *never* do the following, and I understand that these actions would be grounds for discontinuation of my medication therapy:

- Sell or give away my prescriptions or medications

- Forge a prescription

- Steal or borrow another person's medications

- Crush or inject opioid medication

- Use the medication in any way other than prescribed

- Obtain opioid prescription medications from other physicians

- Obtain opioid prescription medication from nonmedical sources

- Use opioid medications with illicit drugs

- Repeatedly lose my prescriptions or medications

- Use multiple pharmacies or the Internet

- Frequently ask you to increase my narcotic medications (for example, because I took more than was prescribed, lost medications, or had it stolen or "accidentally" destroyed)

- Give my medications to someone else

I have the following questions I would like to discuss with you:

- What are your rules for tapering the medication if necessary? If it is determined that I need to taper off the opioid medication, what other pain management approach should or could be added to maximize my pain relief? Will you ask for specialty assistance from another health care provider if necessary?

- Do you have any limitations on prescriptions? What is your policy on the use of break-through pain medications?

- What do I do if I find myself in a pain emergency? Can I call your office? How long can I expect to wait to get a return call from your office? Is pain ever considered an emergency in your practice?

- What are your refill and dose adjustment policies and procedures? Can I ever get my medications early—for example, if I go on a vacation?

- What do we do if things do not work out? What is our exit strategy? Do you agree that the following would indicate that my medication plan is not working?

    1. lack of significant pain reduction as defined by me

    2. lack of improvement in function (my ability to engage in life's activities) or quality of life

    3. continuous negative side effects (such as fatigue, dizziness, nausea, or constipation)

Patient Signature: _____   Physician Signature: _____

Date: _____   Date: _____

TO SUM UP

Now that you understand medication, you are ready to move away from the physical body and on to the psychosocial component of your pain. Remember that your pain is a force connected to every aspect of your life. No one pill or exercise or therapy or skill will change it. Utilizing the comprehensive biopsychosocial model, you have the power of three. This approach will get you where you want to go.

CHAPTER 8

Changing Your Thoughts and Ideas About Chronic Pain

Essentially, in the biopsychosocial model, the psychological component of your pain is the ideas and thoughts you have about living with pain, along with the emotional suffering that often comes with living with a long-term pain problem. The psychological component may be the most important in terms of overall function and quality of life. In fact, some people in pain find vast improvements without changing anything more than their ideas and thoughts about living with pain.

Shakespeare wrote in *Hamlet*, "There is nothing either good or bad, but thinking makes it so" (act 2, scene 2). Perspective is the hinge on which reality hangs. It's also been said that where the mind goes, the body is sure to follow. In some religions, thought is so linked to the physical that sins of thought are as grievous as sins of the flesh. One thing is certain: *how* you think and *what* you think affect what you do, what you feel, and how you interact with others—and all of these affect your pain.

One of the greatest risk factors for ongoing disability and dysfunction from chronic pain is unproductive beliefs, thoughts, and ideas about pain. This chapter will present seven classic ideas you may have developed living with chronic pain and present alternative ways of viewing your pain that may improve the quality of your life.

The chapter will also examine the idea of *self-talk*: the internal conversations and judgments that stream through your mind. There is a direct connection between how you think and how you feel. As you go through life, you take in things that happen around you and evaluate them in a private conversation with yourself. Your self-talk happens so quickly and so automatically that you often react to situations and events before you know that you have evaluated them. Self-talk can determine how you feel and what you choose to do or not to do.

THOUGHTS AND COPING

People react differently to pain. How you cope with your pain is largely based on how functional you are physically and psychologically. The more you are able to do the things you want, the easier it is to cope with pain. The more you are able to view yourself as healthy, the more sound your ideas and thoughts about living with pain. Conversely, the more you see yourself as sick, injured, or damaged, mentally or physically, the harder it is to cope with life. In short, the higher your psychological and physical function, the better you do. Your thoughts and ideas about having pain can play a major role in determining how well or how poorly you cope with pain.

Ellis and Harper (1975) introduced an important way of looking at how thoughts and beliefs influence behavior in their work helping people with problems other than chronic pain. However, many pain management centers around the world have adapted this model to evaluate how people's thoughts and beliefs shape the chronic pain experience.

Ellis and Harper used the phrase "irrational beliefs and dysfunctional thoughts" when they introduced this cognitive behavioral approach. Cognitive behavioral techniques are very helpful for people in pain. However, saying that someone has irrational beliefs and dysfunctional thoughts may be counterproductive, since these words tend to put people off.

Beliefs may be much harder to change than ideas about pain. People tend to defend their beliefs possessively and protectively, as they would their flag or country. When you change your perspective and move from the notion of having "irrational beliefs and dysfunctional thoughts" about living with pain to having "ideas" about living with pain, you make a positive shift toward a more flexible, adaptable, and accepting perspective.

The important consideration about your thoughts and ideas about pain is whether they are working for or against you. Therefore, throughout this chapter, I will be talking about the ideas you have about living with chronic pain, rather than any irrational beliefs and dysfunctional thoughts. A subtle difference, I know, but an important one.

The cognitive behavioral model of changing ideas can be summarized in the acronym ABCD. A stands for the activating event or stressor. An event doesn't have to be physical; it can be an emotional, social, or environmental occurrence, but it is something to which you could have a reaction. For example, the activating event could be a pain flare-up. B stands for the belief (or, as I prefer, idea) that you have about the event. For example, in response to the pain flare-up, you may have the idea that it is awful to suffer from chronic pain. C stands for the consequence of your idea about the event. The consequence is frequently an emotion or feeling state. For example, as a consequence of the idea that living with chronic pain is awful, you might feel anger, resentment, and depression. This ABC pattern typically occurs almost instantaneously, without thought, and you may start to believe that it is instinct, something you cannot influence. But here is where the intervention is launched. D represents an attempt to dispute any falsehoods or errors about your ideas related to the event. Challenging or disputing inaccurate ideas about pain can lead to new feelings and emotions about the event. Later in this chapter, I'll show you how you can do this. But first, let me share a story that illustrates the importance of the last step.

■ John

John was a young man who came to me for help with chronic debilitating migraines. He was a nineteen-year-old college student when he was walking on a bridge between two buildings on campus. It was night, very cold, and he thought no one was around until he heard a commotion below him. Leaning over the railing of the bridge, he saw what appeared to be a homeless man being beaten by two younger men with baseball bats. Transfixed by panic, John watched the homeless man being beaten until he finally stopped moving. Only when the attackers had run away did John break his paralysis and run to the man's side. Though the man was still alive, he was beaten beyond recognition.

John could not stop thinking about the beating. Even after the men were caught, tried, and convicted, he continued to be tormented by the memory. Just like the security videotape that had been used to convict the two men, John kept replaying the events of that night over and over, frame by frame, his guilt growing each time. And just like the security video, John's thoughts stopped when he got to the part where he rolled the man over and saw his horribly beaten face.

John was in terrible emotional pain. He had dropped out of college and was living with his parents. He couldn't work, couldn't sleep, and was plagued by the recurring migraines. All medical reasons for the migraines had been ruled out.

As we discussed what had happened, as John referred again and again to the video and how his memory was just like the videotape, I began to see a way into his guilt, a way to help him out.

"What happened to the man?" I finally asked one day.

John startled and looked blank for a moment. "Oh, um, he spent some time in the hospital."

"How'd he get there?"

"I called 9-1-1."

"And how is he now?"

"Uh, fine. He spent a few days in the hospital and then moved home to Jersey to live with a cousin."

I was stunned, but didn't say so. After all John had said, I was sure the man had died. John had been hitting the pause button whenever he played back his memory of that night, stopping it at the worst moment—the moment when he thought the man would surely die. He never played out the memory to when he saved the man's life, served as a witness during the trial, and learned that the man had gone on with life. He was reliving the negative emotions of the memory but not allowing himself to move past it.

With time and effort, John learned to release the pause button and play the memory to its conclusion. Once he started to allow the memory to complete itself, to go through the beating and the phone call for help and the subsequent trial, his migraines began to subside. He stopped seeing himself as the man who had let another man be beaten and began to believe that maybe he had saved the man's life after all.

John's story is rather extreme, but it's a powerful example of the connections between thoughts, emotions, and pain. The activating event does not have to be traumatic to cause pain. In fact, the events and thoughts we'll focus on in this chapter are your experiences of and ideas about chronic pain. With practice, you can learn to challenge and alter ideas about pain that are causing you emotional distress and compromising your quality of life.

There are seven common ideas or thought patterns people tend to develop when they live with chronic pain:

1. Catastrophizing

2. Fear of reinjury

3. Expectation of a cure

4. Entitlement, frustration, and anger

5. Self-blame

6. Future despair

7. Social disbelief

We are going to examine each and consider which ideas have become problems in your life—problems that may exacerbate and maintain your pain experience.

Your job (and I'm here to help) is to modify any unhelpful or unhealthy ideas and thoughts you have about your pain. My experience and research have taught me that by challenging unproductive ideas about chronic pain, people can lead a better life and can function at a more acceptable level.

CATASTROPHIZING

Earlier in this book, I discussed the concept of pain flare-ups and the notion that pain is a series of time-limited flare-ups instead of an all-encompassing, never-ending experience. Your ideas about pain can be triggers that initiate, worsen, or even maintain a pain flare-up.

Catastrophizing about pain often takes the form of thoughts like:

This pain is awful. I will be stuck with this pain forever.

I can't stand this pain. What if my pain never gets better? My future is shot.

If I have this kind of pain now, it is going to get worse, and it will be terrible by the evening.

> *Fear is that little darkroom where negatives are developed.*
>
> —Michael Prichard

Catastrophizing happens when you take one piece of information (*I hurt*) and conclude that everything else will be awful and terrible. You blow the anticipated experience way out of proportion, to the point that you become miserable. This thought pattern also reflects the idea that it is awful and catastrophic when things don't go the way you want them to.

Catastrophic thinking is certainly understandable. One idea builds on another, reinforcing a host of other negative ideas and creating a vortex of negativity. This exaggerated negativity about pain can be as hard to escape as a tornado—and as damaging. Catastrophic thinking is a stress-producing process that perpetuates pain.

When you start thinking in a catastrophic way, you come to so expect the negative that you brace yourself for it even if it never comes. You worry about negative consequences so much that you start to expect the worst from even minor events. Your thoughts are dominated by this rumination, by your magnified reactions, to the point where you feel helpless and out of control of your life. Pain becomes a self-fulfilling prophecy. And even if you are not happy, you take comfort in the fact that you can predict the future, which offers some kind of control. This sense of control is the real attraction of catastrophic thinking.

The tendency toward catastrophic thinking is an accurate predictor of the intensity of physical and emotional distress experienced by people in pain. It is a kind of measurement of a person's ability (or, actually, inability) to clearly see a situation. Catastrophizing creates a smudge on the lens through which you see your life. As you continue catastrophizing, as your tendency becomes an actual prophecy, that smudge grows and thickens until you are incapable of seeing a situation clearly. Instead, you simply assume.

Let's start by looking at some of the ideas you may have about living with pain. Take this quick survey.

EXERCISE 8.1: CATASTROPHIC IDEAS SCALE

How strongly do you agree or disagree with the following statements?

My pain problem is more than I can handle.

strongly disagree						strongly agree	
0	1	2	3	4	5	6	7

I can get on with the business of living despite my pain.

strongly disagree						strongly agree	
0	1	2	3	4	5	6	7

I am in control of my life even though I have pain.

strongly disagree						strongly agree	
0	1	2	3	4	5	6	7

To score this survey, add up the numbers you circled for the last two items and subtract that from 14. Add the score for the first item, then divide by 3. This is your catastrophizing score. This number should be between 0 and 7. Add your score to your Pain Scorecard at the end of this book.

Interpreting Your Score

Level three: 3.7 or more.   If you score at this level, you tend to magnify the threat of your pain. You may feel you are incapable of dealing with pain, that the pain is awful and terrible, and that pain controls your life.

Level two: 2.0 to 3.6.   You are similar to most people who suffer from chronic pain. You may believe that your pain is in the driver's seat while you ride in the back—or worse, the trunk—with little or no control. You may think things like *I will be stuck in this pain forever* or *Having pain means I have nothing to look forward to.*

Level one: 1.9 or less.   Congratulations. Your score is less than the majority of chronic pain patients. You are likely handling your pain fairly well and are not catastrophizing about your pain and letting it control your life. You are probably not jumping to conclusions or assuming the worst when you experience your pain.

If you find yourself in level two or three, you need to begin working on your core ideas about living with chronic pain.

The Effects of Catastrophizing

Catastrophizing is more than a head game you play with yourself. It has a profound effect on your emotions, your relationships, and your experience of physical distress.

Catastrophizing and Chronic Pain

The cycle of catastrophic ideas about pain causes a cycle of behaviors that can maintain and intensify chronic pain. If you are always expecting to be in pain, always looking for the pain, you will notice your pain more, and thus it will be worse.

One reason people catastrophize about their pain is that they misinterpret bodily sensations as evidence that something is seriously wrong physically. An ambiguous situation arises (for example, you feel a painful sensation and you don't know the cause) and you experience the situation as a catastrophic event that is directly related to your physical problems. Anxiety and worry follow, and you begin to feel out of control of your life.

Repeatedly engaging in catastrophic thinking can lead you to develop enduring beliefs that painful stimuli are always significant and threatening and that you are unable to effectively manage the stress associated with painful experiences. Whether or not these thoughts are based on truth, they change how you live.

Catastrophizing and Relationships

If you find yourself catastrophizing about your pain and also rate your pain in the upper third of the pain intensity scale, you are more likely to experience significant limitations on your social life. My own research backs this up. People with this combination see friends and relatives less often, go out less, and travel less. The fear of pain begins to rule their lives. But it's not just a matter of fear. Women who rate their pain in the upper third of the pain scale and who catastrophize about their pain also have less energy. Catastrophizing hits those in pain mentally, physically, and socially—a trifecta of perpetual disability.

People who engage in a lot of catastrophic thinking often have a high need for emotional support from others. Asking for what you want and need straightforwardly and honestly is a critical pain management skill. Poor communication skills, an inability to ask for what you want and need, leads to a passive and unassertive style of interaction. Learning assertiveness skills provides a means of asking for what you need—and increases your chances of getting it. (I'll say more about assertiveness in chapter 11.)

Persistence of Anxiety

Don't get down on yourself if you find that you have catastrophic ideas about your pain. Negative and catastrophic interpretations of health information are common. The majority of people are liable to occasionally become briefly preoccupied with unexplained bodily variations. However, such episodes of health anxiety usually go away. Your symptoms fade, you absorb reassuring information from a doctor with relief (if you believe the information), and the anxiety about your health declines and disappears. If your health anxiety does not fade, or if it escalates to the point of dominating your life, you need to work to understand what it is that causes the anxiety to persist.

It is the persistence of anxiety that creates a vicious cycle. We will discuss many such vicious cycles of pain in this book. Catastrophizing, subsequent anxiety, and pain is just one of them.

Catastrophizing and Heightened Levels of Distress

Examining the extent of your catastrophizing is useful in measuring your susceptibility to heightened distress responses to pain. Knowing your degree or level of catastrophic thinking will help you find the coping interventions that will be most effective in promoting your recovery from pain.

People who catastrophize about their pain usually have an exaggerated negative orientation toward pain. Now, few of us hold a very positive outlook on being in pain. But when you catastrophize, you exaggerate the threat value of your pain. You will tend to believe in the worst and fail to consider other possibilities about having pain.

Modifying Catastrophic Thinking

So what do you do? How do you change catastrophic ideas about having pain? Is it possible to learn positive or useful ideas and thoughts about your pain?

Because catastrophizing is controlled by you, you are able to alter it. The key is to modify your thinking. In this section, I'll offer some strategies to help you modify your thoughts, your internal dialog, and thus the ideas you have about your pain experience. But keep in mind that you alone can determine what works for you. You may want to try a variety of strategies; mix and match at will. Pay attention to what works for you and what doesn't. Feel free to customize the suggestions to suit your temperament, your experience, and your life. No one strategy is better than another, although having choices is empowering in coping with chronic pain.

Critically Evaluate Your Thoughts

The first strategy is to look at how accurate and realistic your ideas are about having pain and challenge them as ideas and assumptions rather than indisputable facts. I want you to think of yourself as a scientist or a researcher, someone who sets out hypotheses about pain and then tests them to see if they are accurate. I will not tell you what to think or how to think; rather, I'll guide you in making discoveries about yourself and your pain.

EXERCISE 8.2: THOUGHT EVALUATION FORM

Judith Beck (1996) has created a worksheet to evaluate unproductive ideas about living with chronic pain. Below is her worksheet, the Thought Evaluation Form, which I believe is very helpful for people suffering from chronic pain.

Thought Evaluation Form

Automatic thought:

What is the evidence that the automatic thought is true?

What is the evidence that the automatic thought is not true?

Is there an alternative explanation?

What is the worst that could happen if the automatic thought were true? Could I live with it?

What's the best that could happen?

What is the most realistic outcome?

What's the effect of my believing the automatic thought? (advantages/disadvantages of believing it)

What could be the effect of changing my thinking? (advantages/disadvantages of letting go of it)

What should I do about it?

If _____ (friend's name) were in this situation, what would I tell him/her?

MATTHEW'S THOUGHT EVALUATION FORM

Matthew was a forty-five-year-old married man who had low back pain for several years as the result of a lifting accident at work. His life had changed dramatically, and he was only a shell of the man he had been before his injury. He was no longer able to go camping with his family, and he felt guilty about not working. Because of pain, he was experiencing depression and sleep problems.

Here is how he filled out the Thought Evaluation Form.

Automatic thought:

I will never be able to get on with my life with this pain. This pain is more than I can handle.

What is the evidence that the automatic thought is true?

When I wake up in the morning, my pain is killing me, and I get frustrated that it hasn't gone away, and I feel sad. I start feeling depressed. I don't know if I can go on with this.

What is the evidence that the automatic thought is not true?

I have had some times (although not many) when I felt okay and had some fun (at a birthday party, seeing a funny movie) even though I had pain.

Is there an alternative explanation?

Pain is tough to live with, but it is possible that if I learn some new relaxation skills like deep breathing, I will feel better and be more in control of my pain.

What is the worst that could happen if the automatic thought were true? Could I live with it?

Never being able to be happy is a depressing thought, and I would be miserable and not fun to be around. You know, I am already living with it, so I guess I could live with it, but I don't like it!

What's the best that could happen?

The best thing that could happen if I ended up never being happy is that maybe my family and doctors would finally realize that my pain is serious and real and try to find some treatment or something that would help me.

What is the most realistic outcome?

Well, I guess I will continue to explore other ways of coping with my pain and maybe focus on those times when I have fun. Since I have had some fun in the past, I guess I can try to have more good times, even with this pain.

What's the effect of my believing the automatic thought? (advantages/disadvantages of believing it)

By believing that I will never be happy as long as I have pain, I guess I have an excuse to be miserable. The disadvantage of believing this idea is that others don't want to be around me because I am such a downer. The advantage may be that sometimes I don't want others around, and I use the pain as an excuse to be alone.

What could be the effect of changing my thinking? (advantages/disadvantages of letting go of it)

I guess the main advantage of changing my way of thinking about happiness and pain is that they don't have to be mutually exclusive. I can have pain and still be somewhat happy. One doesn't have to control the other. The main disadvantage of letting go of the idea is that I would have to work at it, and that takes energy.

What should I do about it?

I need to start realizing that happiness is not an all-or-nothing emotion and that happiness has varying degrees. It is not an absolute thing. I also need to realize that people who do not have pain can also be unhappy. I know that I need to learn to start taking a more active role in managing my pain. I can't wait for others to do something for me to be happier—I have to do it.

If Sally were in this situation, what would I tell her?

If my friend Sally were in my situation, I would try to help her see that attitude is an important part of any experience and that ideas that are all or nothing or black and white don't seem to be realistic and helpful.

Find Evidence of Control

As you critically evaluate your ideas, you'll begin to see that there are some things you can control and some things you can't. Feeling a sense of control over your pain is empowering. At the same time, you cannot totally control whether or not you're going to have pain. You can control how you choose to interpret your pain sensations and how you respond to them. It is all about coping and managing pain rather than curing and eliminating it.

Get Input from Others

Because it may be difficult to assess your own thoughts, talk to your family members and friends. Ask them to monitor and record your actions (how often you talk about how bad your pain is, how well you get on with life, how often you do normal things). Consider how your actions—as others see them—reflect your thoughts.

You can also gain perspective on your own thoughts by learning how others think. You might interview members of a pain support group and ask how they think about and cope with pain.

Remember That Hurt Does Not Mean Harm

The ability to separate hurt from harm can be a critical strategy for coping with pain. By definition, all pain hurts, but unlike acute pain, chronic pain is not a reliable indicator of harm. If you believe that you have experienced harm, you need medical attention. But not all pain necessarily means that you have suffered harm or need medical attention. Learn to discriminate between an intensification of the same old pain and a totally new sensation or pain in a new location. If you experience a new and different sensation in a new physical location, it needs attention.

Use Expressive Writing

Writing is a beneficial coping strategy for some people with chronic pain. Expressive writing has led to less disability and improved mood for people who score high on the Catastrophic Ideas Scale. Long-term suppression of intense emotions frequently leads to increased stress, which has negative effects including compromised immune function. Living with chronic pain can easily be seen as a long-term stressor, and providing an outlet for the intense emotions related to living with chronic pain can help reduce stress.

EXERCISE 8.3: EXPRESSIVE WRITING

Consider writing in a journal your thoughts and feelings as you experience a major pain flare-up or anticipate an upcoming medical procedure. Focus on the aspects you find most distressing. Your notes are only for you, so don't worry about editing or censoring your thoughts. This exercise can help you clarify and understand your feelings related to pain.

Reinterpret Pain Sensations

Taking a slightly different perspective on your pain sensations can change their effect. Try completing the following sentences:

The pain I am now experiencing is a sign of _____ *(normal soreness, overdoing it, staying in one position too long, and so on).*

The pain is a signal that I could practice my _____ *(breathing exercises, relaxation skills, and so on).*

This pain I feel now is likely due to _____ *(muscle tension, bracing myself too long, and so on).*

Divert Your Attention

Think of your attention as a flashlight beam in a dark room. Focus your attention on an area of your body where pain sensations are absent. Redirecting attention to external activities can also help reduce your pain awareness. You could engage in some physical or mental activity like doing a crossword puzzle, playing a video game, or reading. Divert your attention to a pleasant memory from a time prior to the onset of your pain.

Use Positive Coping Statements

When you find yourself catastrophizing, consider using positive coping statements:

My life is not determined by pain but by . . .

It is not critical that I control the pain. It's about managing and coping.

This pain flare-up will only last for . . .

I have the ability to . . .

I can stay active by . . .

FEAR OF REINJURY

Now that we've thoroughly addressed catastrophizing, let's take a look at another idea common among people who live with chronic pain: fear of reinjury. To begin, take this survey.

EXERCISE 8.4: FEAR OF REINJURY SCALE

How strongly do you agree or disagree with the following statements?

When I do things that increase my pain, I am concerned that I might reinjure myself.

strongly disagree   strongly agree
0   1   2   3   4   5   6   7

The best way to cope with chronic pain is by resting and avoiding those activities that make the pain worse.

strongly disagree   strongly agree
0   1   2   3   4   5   6   7

If I exert myself physically, I am only asking for trouble, since I could reinjure myself.

strongly disagree   strongly agree
0   1   2   3   4   5   6   7

To score this exercise, add up all the numbers you circled, then divide the result by 3. This is your fear of reinjury score. This number should be between 0 and 7. Place it in the Pain Scorecard.

Interpreting Your Score

Level three: 5.1 or more.   Your level of fear of reinjury places you in the upper third of people with chronic pain. Fear of reinjury is a significant problem in your day-to-day life. Fear of reinjury and fear of movement in general explains how other negative ideas about pain—in particular, catastrophic interpretations of a pain flare-up—can lead to avoidance of movement and activities. This negative feedback cycle contributes to maintaining and exacerbating fear, disuse, emotional distress, and dysfunction.

Level two: 3.2 to 5.0.   You are in the middle range compared with most other people living with chronic pain. Chances are, you are fearful that engaging in physical activities may result in increased pain and possible injury. You have likely adopted a strategy of avoiding many activities. Your scores on the activity avoidance scales in chapter 10 are also likely to be moderate to high. If so, then life is probably passing you by because of pain.

Level one: 3.1 or less.   Fear of reinjury may not be a significant area of concern for your pain treatment strategy. You're not likely worried and fearful of reinjuring yourself, and you're not likely avoiding a lot of activities. In chapter 10, I'll present a series of activity interference and activity avoidance scales. Low scores on these scales would verify that you are not avoiding many activities of daily living.

Disability and Fear of Reinjury

Dealing with chronic pain is a challenge. There's no two ways about it. And most people will do whatever they can to avoid it. While there is nothing inherently wrong with trying to avoid pain, the problem sneaks in when you let the avoidance of pain alter your thoughts and take over your life. Hypervigilance replaces common sense; fear replaces care.

Gordon Waddell, a prominent medical researcher in the field of pain, once said, "Fear of pain and what we do about it is more disabling than the pain itself." Waddell and colleagues (1993) found that the best predictor of return to work after a reported back injury was the worker's beliefs about what would happen to their symptoms and their body upon return to work. The degree of anticipation of reinjury was more predictive of return to work than the presence or severity of symptoms. The same is likely true for those who suffer from other pain types and return to productive life other than work.

In fact, *fear-avoidance* patterns (avoiding activities because you are afraid of being reinjured) can lead to persistent disability. This is especially true in people with back pain. The belief and expectation that activity will cause injury makes the pain worse. As the pain becomes worse, the avoidance becomes stronger, until a person is virtually bedridden by both fear and physical deconditioning.

Some Hard Truths About Fear of Reinjury

Many researchers, including Buer and Linton (2002), suggest that fear-avoidance beliefs and catastrophic thinking about pain are critical in driving the transition from acute to chronic pain.

High fears of reinjury invoke high feelings of anxiety and worry that activity will make things worse. If you scored high on the Fear of Reinjury Scale, try to think how you got there. Why are you afraid of hurting yourself? Have you actually reinjured yourself before? Has something a doctor said scared you? I've seen clients who come in with chronic pain that they are afraid will turn to paralysis if they move wrong. Often, this is because of a warning from a doctor. Unfortunately, these well-heeded warnings frequently scare people into a life of inactivity and fear.

Some people believe that if something is fearsome, dangerous, or unpleasant (like pain), they should be terribly concerned about it and dwell on the possibility that it will occur. This is a stress-producing idea. Anxiety and worry may hamper your ability to cope with other real-life situations and events. Extreme concern often leads to exaggerated fantasies about the potential harm of a situation that actually have no basis in fact. If you hold these ideas, it will likely be reflected in your experience of fear, hopelessness, anxiety, and avoidance.

Overcoming Fear of Reinjury

Here are some things you can do if you scored at level two or three on the Fear of Reinjury Scale.

Confront your fear with realistic information and exposure to graduated movement and exercise. Ask your physician about your diagnosis and your pain generators. Having a realistic notion of what is causing your pain can greatly reduce your fears. Ask your physical therapist if it is possible for you to gravely hurt yourself with movement activities. Chances are you can't, but you may need that reassurance to know it is safe to resume some activities.

You may be helped by seeing a physical therapist who understands chronic pain issues—someone who can help you with activity pacing. Massage, rest, and heat help in the short term but not in the long run. When you choose a therapist, avoid any that preach or even imply "no pain, no gain." Many people report therapy makes their pain worse. If that is because the therapist pushed them, then the therapist is a problem. But the problem also might be unrealistic fears of reinjury. Find a comfortable match with a therapist who respects your condition but also has the power to guide you in returning to normal function.

Avoiding activity means your world will shrink, which frequently leads to isolation. Odds are, you will become indecisive, immobilized, and prone to procrastinate. Activity pacing and learning to break unhelpful associations (such as *The more I do, the more I hurt*) will help address your fears of reinjury.

Go back to exercise 4.6, your Pain Flare-Up Record, to see if you checked any fear of reinjury ideas under the psychological trigger section. If so, what was the pain flare-up situation, and what level of anxiety did you have during that flare-up? You can continue to use the Pain Flare-Up Record to validate your success in reducing your endorsement of these ideas related to future pain flare-ups.

Reduce anxiety and fears by practicing relaxation skills such as breathing and meditation. High fears of reinjury are frequently associated with muscle tension, guarding, and bracing behaviors. Use the blue dots discussed in exercise 6.2 as a reminder to let go of excess tension and practice deep diaphragmatic breathing.

EXERCISE 8.5: TRACK YOUR PAIN INTENSITY AND FEAR OF REINJURY

Track your fear of reinjury scores and pain levels using this graph. By tracking the Fear of Reinjury Scale frequently, you may begin to see how illogical some of your ideas about reinjury are in reference to your day-to-day pain experience.

PAIN INTENSITY AND FEAR OF REINJURY

Treatment: _____

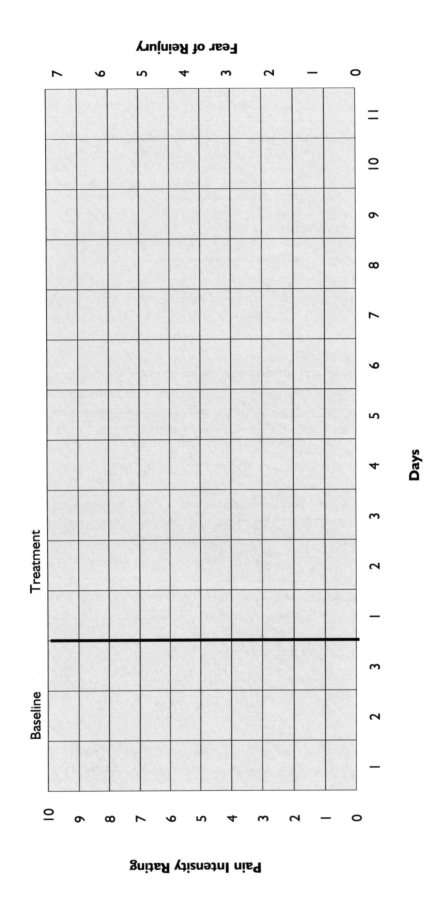

EXPECTATION OF A CURE

Living with chronic pain in a world seemingly filled with healthy people and health care miracles, you can develop unreasonable (although understandable) expectations. Ideas about being cured or fixed—ideas of having your pain eliminated with the right doctor, drug, or surgery—are normal and natural. But they may not be helpful, especially if you have entered the world of chronic pain. Remember that chronic pain may not be a symptom of some underlying, ongoing tissue damage or chronic disease. Unlike acute pain, which provides a useful signal that some tissue injury or damage may need immediate attention, chronic pain frequently does not serve a useful warning function.

Before you read any further, consider how strongly you agree or disagree with the following statement:

I have accepted that nothing further can be done to eliminate my pain.

Most people do not accept that nothing more can be done to treat their pain, and this is very understandable. People work hard at being hopeful. Being hopeful that some medical advancement might ease pain is very important psychologically, because it offers the possibility of something good. Keep some degree of hope and faith. Hope is important for people with chronic pain.

However, the other side of this statement—agreeing that there may not be anything that can be done to eliminate your pain—does not necessarily mean giving up all hope for future improvements in our ability to medically address chronic pain. Rather, it is more about being realistic about what's available today. I frequently use the analogy that you have one hundred eggs in your basket of life. I strongly recommend that you take ten to fifteen of those eggs and put them in the basket called "hope"—hope that new technologies will come along in the future to reduce pain and suffering. But I also strongly recommend that you keep the other eighty-five to ninety eggs in the basket of living today. Unrealistic expectation of a cure or fix for your pain can rob you of living in the now.

■ *Amanda*

Amanda, who suffered from a herniated cervical disk, was my first client who had had an artificial disk replacement. To me, she was a medical novelty. She had waited a long time for this surgery, which had only recently been sanctioned by the American Medical Association. Amanda's expectations were very high, and she expected to be pain-free following the surgery.

Unfortunately, Amanda had been doing many things that were counterproductive from a pain management perspective. She had been taking her time-released pain medications as needed, not at specific time intervals. She let pain be her guide and frequently stayed in bed for hours, getting little to no exercise. When she did get out of bed, she would overdo activities, until pain forced her back into bed. Prior to the surgery, she said that she expected 100 percent pain relief from the procedure, or it would be a failure. The stage was set for disaster.

Five months following the surgery, Amanda's neck pain was as bad as it ever had been, and she was angry, frustrated, and depressed. When I asked what she thought was currently causing her pain, she stated firmly that "a piece of my neck is missing" and that this was terrible and awful. Her unrealistic expectations, coupled with unproductive pain management strategies, led her right into my office.

On a positive note, we were able to work on developing realistic expectations and addressed the secondary problems she was having—including reframing the way she thought about her body—and she did improve. Having some positive expectations is healthy, but having unrealistic expectations frequently perpetuates the chronic pain experience.

ENTITLEMENT, FRUSTRATION, AND ANGER

Let's take a close look at another set of ideas and emotions experienced by many who suffer from chronic pain: entitlement, frustration, and anger. To begin, complete this exercise. Your entitlement/frustration score is a reflection of the toll that anger and frustration have taken on your life.

EXERCISE 8.6: ENTITLEMENT/FRUSTRATION SCALE

How strongly do you agree or disagree with the following statements?

It isn't right that I'm experiencing chronic pain.

strongly disagree						strongly agree	
0	1	2	3	4	5	6	7

I shouldn't have to suffer from this pain.

strongly disagree						strongly agree	
0	1	2	3	4	5	6	7

I deserve better than to have chronic pain.

strongly disagree						strongly agree	
0	1	2	3	4	5	6	7

To score this exercise, add up the numbers you circled, then divide by 3. This is your entitlement/frustration score. This number should be between 0 and 7. Add it to your Pain Scorecard.

Interpreting Your Score

Level three: 5.5 or more.   Entitlement and frustration is a major area of concern. You are probably saying to yourself, *Why me? Why do I have this pain problem? It's not fair that I have this pain.* In my research using the BAP questionnaire, I found that entitlement/frustration was the second-highest average score for this section, suggesting that most people who suffer from chronic pain are angry at having to live with pain. This scale also correlates highly with depression, worry that you will not be productive in your daily life, and fear of pain.

Level two: 4.3 to 5.4.   Your score is within the typical range for the majority of people who have chronic pain. You are moderately affected by anger and frustration.

Level one: 4.2 or less.   If you scored at this level, you have minimal difficulty with anger issues compared to most people with chronic pain. This may be considered a strength in your pain self-management program. Perhaps you have become annoyed with your pain, but you have not let this feeling get out of control and dominate your life.

Discomfort and pain are normal parts of life. Just ask anyone over fifty. Chances are, they have some pain just from the aging process. If you begin to believe that you shouldn't have any discomfort or pain and that it is your right to feel good, you will develop problems—problems with expectations that are unrealistic.

Unmet expectations often lead to the frustrating feeling that you are entitled to feel better than you do. The frustration of entitlement slips easily into anger, so let's start there and work our way back.

Anger

While much of the research about pain and mood-related problems has focused on depression and anxiety, it has been my experience that anger is perhaps the greatest stumbling block to physical and emotional recovery and wellness. Here are some of the many factors that contribute to anger:

- The relentlessness of chronic pain

- Treatment failures

- Pain experienced as a result of treatments

- Invalidation of the pain experience by others (physicians, employers, insurance companies, family, and friends)

Anger is strongly associated with the amount of pain you experience and how much it stops you from doing what it is you want to do. Anger isn't necessarily a bad emotion. It's a legitimate reaction. But the heightened arousal that comes with high levels of anger exacerbates pain. So, how you deal with anger is critical to your pain experience and to your level of motivation for engaging in treatment.

Anger is associated with a variety of negative health consequences, including high blood pressure, cardiac arrhythmias, and stroke. It is therefore not surprising that anger significantly affects the experience of pain as well. Anger is an emotion, but its impact is physical as well. Anger can change how your body responds, and it can change how you behave.

The negative functions of anger include confusing thoughts, negative thoughts, and aggression. It can also drive other people away, possibly setting the stage for isolation. Anger can make you frustrated, irritable, and cynical. Anger can lead you to focus on the negative characteristics of your pain over all else, clouding your judgment with overgeneralizations and false conclusions.

Not only does the mere experience of anger appear to affect responses to pain; so too does the way you manage your anger. There are two primary ways people manage anger: by turning it inward (suppressing anger) and by turning it outward (expressing anger verbally or physically). Both are associated with sensitivity to both acute and chronic pain.

The consequences of anger are not entirely negative. Anger does serve some positive functions as well. Anger can be an energizer; it can make you feel in control, a feeling pain has taken away from many people. This is why so many people in pain are angry—in part, because anger can lead to a perceived sense of control. The problem is that unaddressed and unabated anger gets in the way of healing and impedes your ability to manage your own pain rehabilitation.

Entitlement and Frustration

Entitlement usually centers around the idea that it is not fair for you to be in pain and that you don't deserve pain. The key word is "fair." There is nothing fair about chronic pain. No one deserves chronic pain. Chronic pain is not a punishment for being a bad person. Whether you think your pain is from an injury, clumsiness, karma, or just plain bad luck, you can make your experience better.

Regardless of why or how you think your pain is unfair, the idea of entitlement (believing the situation should be different because it's unfair) goes hand in hand with blame, frustration, and anger. It is easy to get stuck in these emotions and stop moving forward. The danger is that your thoughts will always be on these concepts of fairness rather than on improving your experience with pain. Many people with high levels of blame, frustration, and anger stop moving and stop improving. They don't get better. Anger, blame, and frustration take up space in your head, which doesn't leave much room for anything else. Don't give these emotions free rent in your head.

■ Chuck

Chuck was forty-two when he got sideswiped by a drunk driver. His injuries were extensive, but the worst for him was the loss of his right leg. Phantom pain served as a constant reminder of the accident. *Why me?* had become such a repetitive thought for him that it was like a song he couldn't get out of his mind. After two years of near-constant pain, he came to me to see if there was something he could be doing to feel better. After taking the BAP, he found that the problem was not so much the physical injury as his thoughts and ideas about losing his leg.

In all my years treating people with chronic pain, I have never seen such high entitlement scores as Chuck's. Chuck was so frustrated and so angry and had been for so long that he didn't even recognize it anymore. When he talked, his voice rose, and he quickly became agitated. He had not done anything to deserve being hit by a drunk driver. He was a good man who always obeyed the rules. The driver of the SUV that hit him had run a red light and even left the scene of the accident (leaving Chuck pinned in his totaled Camry), only to be caught three blocks later when he ran into a light pole. The driver wasn't even bruised. It wasn't fair.

When Chuck saw his entitlement scores, his first reaction was "But it wasn't my fault." I agreed with him. It wasn't fair that this accident had befallen him. But that didn't change the indisputable fact that it had happened. The guy who hit him wasn't going to give his leg back or take away the pain; he'd never even apologized. Nobody was going to come along and say, "Oh, we didn't realize. You're right. This is unfair. Let me fix it." Chuck knew this logically, but he hadn't really accepted it.

Over time and with some work, starting with coming to terms with that BAP score, Chuck began to let go of his anger and entitlement. As he did, he freed space in his mind for some new ideas. I continually reminded him that the people who successfully manage their pain are those who are successful at diffusing entitlement, frustration, and anger. They know how to let the steam out and not dwell on the unfairness of the situation. We worked on replacing *Why me?* with more productive thoughts. Chuck found that he could ease his frustration just by telling himself, *I may not like the pain, but I am doing the best I can* and *By blaming others, I just get myself more upset, and that comes back to make me feel worse.*

As he concentrated on releasing his resentment and even moved toward forgiving the drunk driver (not because the driver deserved forgiveness, but because Chuck deserved to be rid of his anger), Chuck's rehab began to improve. His pain lessened, his anger dissipated, and old friends who had been avoiding him started coming around again. Chuck still had pain, but he felt better, and feeling better is no small accomplishment.

Anger and entitlement are major obstacles to any kind of recovery. My experience has been that those people who most effectively address their anger and entitlement do the best in rehabilitation.

The Power of Words

Empowerment is the opposite of entitlement. If you are reeling from toxic thoughts and feelings of entitlement and anger, you need to free space in your mind. Finding a sense of empowerment is the quickest way to free that space. The simplest form of empowerment is in the power of words.

A sense of guilt or obligation is often associated with the word "should" (or its cousin "must"). Get rid of this word, and instead, use the word "could." The word "could" empowers you and gives you a choice, which in turn allows you to take credit for your actions. Thinking in terms of "should" can lead to depression and make you feel at fault. This will only further distance you from empowerment.

Another unproductive and overused word is "can't." Try replacing "can't" with "won't." With "can't" you feel immobilized, hopeless, and helpless. With "won't" you are expressing a decision. "Won't" suggests free choice and the power of options. Using "can't" magnifies or exaggerates a negative event. Such magnification is a distortion of the truth. Feel the difference between these two statements:

I can't stand this pain anymore and can't get on with my life.

I won't stand this pain anymore and won't get on with my life.

The second sentence probably makes you more uncomfortable, even though it is further from the truth. You have a choice about how you live your life. Using "can't" takes that choice away. Take it back.

Other words you might want to banish from your vocabulary are "fix," "cure," "finish," and "eliminate." These words can keep you stuck in your pain patterns because you are holding out too much hope of things changing. They may not. So instead, think about words like "cope," "manage," and "deal." That way, things may change, but you won't be just waiting around—you'll be actively participating in improving your pain experience.

SELF-BLAME

Wanting to be more in control of your pain is normal. Pain often makes you feel like you are in the backseat of life and pain is in the driver's seat. Frequently, people tell me that they feel they should be doing a better job of controlling or coping with their pain. This feeling is common among people who suffer from chronic pain.

Let's take a look at this idea and see how you score.

EXERCISE 8.7: SELF-BLAME SCALE

How strongly do you agree or disagree with the following statements?

I should be able to control the pain much better than I do.

strongly disagree						strongly agree	
0	1	2	3	4	5	6	7

I shouldn't let the pain bother me as much as it does.

strongly disagree						strongly agree	
0	1	2	3	4	5	6	7

I must be doing something wrong since I continue to have pain.

strongly disagree						strongly agree	
0	1	2	3	4	5	6	7

I'm upset with myself for not being able to control my pain better.

strongly disagree						strongly agree	
0	1	2	3	4	5	6	7

To score this exercise, add up all the numbers you circled, then divide the result by 4. This is your self-blame score. This number should be between 0 and 7. Place it on your Pain Scorecard.

Interpreting Your Score

Level three: 3.5 or more.   Your level of self-blame places you in the upper third of people with chronic pain. You are probably beating yourself up about your inability to control your pain and its negative impact on your life and your relations with others. High self-blame scores are associated with catastrophic thinking, depression, and loss of productivity. You may be inclined to have feelings of inferiority, worthlessness, and disappointment with yourself. Self-blame is frequently associated with the unproductive emotion of guilt and the unhelpful word "should."

It is very important to realize that your ideas about pain are just that: ideas. They may or may not be accurate or true. Just because you endorse these ideas does not mean that they are correct or accurate. Learning to argue with yourself and dispute faulty ideas is a key coping strategy for living with pain. Remember to ask yourself, *What is the evidence that this idea is true?*

Level two: 1.8 to 3.4.   You are in the average or middle range compared to most other people with chronic pain. This means self-blame is a part of your life, but it isn't a significant problem.

Level one: 1.7 or less.   You are not likely blaming yourself for not being able to control your pain better. Self-blame may not be a significant area of concern for your pain management. Good job.

FUTURE DESPAIR

Living with pain and its chronic nature can lead to a sense that you will never be happy or have pleasure in your life. A profound sense that there is no hope given a life with pain is by definition depressing. Too often, the future looks nothing but uncertain to people in pain.

This exercise will give you a better understanding of how you see your future.

EXERCISE 8.8: FUTURE DESPAIR SCALE

How strongly do you agree or disagree with the following statements?

I will never enjoy life again as long as I have pain.

	strongly disagree					strongly agree	
0	1	2	3	4	5	6	7

My life will never be filled as long as I have pain.

	strongly disagree					strongly agree	
0	1	2	3	4	5	6	7

I will never be completely happy as long as I have pain.

	strongly disagree					strongly agree	
0	1	2	3	4	5	6	7

To score this exercise, add up all the numbers you circled, then divide by 3. This is your future despair score. This number should be between 0 and 7. Place it on your Pain Scorecard.

Interpreting Your Score

Level three: 3.5 or more. Unhappiness is a major part of your chronic pain experience. As you can imagine, a high future despair score correlates highly with depression. It is also an example of all-or-nothing thinking. A score of 3.5 or higher indicates that future despair is a major area of concern in your pain self-management program.

Level two: 1.4 to 3.4. Your score is within the typical range for the majority of people who have chronic pain. You may have difficulty with depression as a consequence of your chronic pain experience.

Level one: 1.3 or less. Scoring at this level suggests that you have minimal difficulty with unhappiness about your future with pain. This may be considered a strength in your self-management of pain.

Your future despair score is a reflection of the notion that happiness will only come into your life when the pain is gone. With this notion comes the idea that as long as you have any pain, there is no hope that you'll have any positive experiences. Psychological distress results from this idea, captured by the themes of helplessness and hopelessness. If a certain condition is met (having pain), then a certain consequence is expected (never being happy).

A first step in challenging and modifying this idea is to recognize that it is just an idea and not a fact. Ask yourself what experiences you have had that do not fit the idea that you will never be happy as long as you have pain. What is the evidence against this idea? When were you last happy? What were you doing? Chances are, you have been discounting the times when you have experienced something positive.

SOCIAL DISBELIEF

Just because your pain is invisible doesn't mean it's not real. Pain is very real. Even pain from a limb that is no longer there is real. Pain is an experience in the brain, not in the injured body part, as you learned in chapter 2. Unfortunately, not everyone is familiar with the gate-control model or the biopsychosocial perspective. Nor can other people crawl into your brain and feel your pain. So for many people out there, "invisible" means "not real." And if you are in pain and you must deal with these people, this can be a problem.

Let's take a look at your responses to the questions on the Social Disbelief Scale to see how you feel about others' perceptions of your pain.

EXERCISE 8.9: SOCIAL DISBELIEF SCALE

How strongly do you agree or disagree with the following statements?

I sometimes feel I have to show others I am in pain; otherwise, they won't believe my pain is real.

strongly disagree						strongly agree	
0	1	2	3	4	5	6	7

It bothers me that others might not believe my pain is real.

strongly disagree						strongly agree	
0	1	2	3	4	5	6	7

I sometimes feel I have to prove to others that I really do hurt.

strongly disagree						strongly agree	
0	1	2	3	4	5	6	7

To score this exercise, add up all the numbers you circled, then divide the result by 3. This is your social disbelief score. This number should be between 0 and 7. Place your score on your Pain Scorecard.

Interpreting Your Score

Your social disbelief score is a reflection of the extent to which you believe that others don't believe your pain is real or think that you are exaggerating your pain for some gain.

Level three: 2.4 or more.   Social disbelief is a major area of concern in your pain self-management program. It is very likely that you have felt invalidated by some person or entity in your life. Perhaps no one intended to invalidate you; nonetheless, you are reporting that there are people out there who do not believe your experience of pain is as bad as you say it is. Frequently, the disbelieving entity is an institution, like the workers' compensation insurance system if you are an injured worker, or it could be your employer. Sometimes people feel invalidated in their pain complaints by members of the health care system. This is particularly bad when it is your treating physician, nurse, or therapist. Closer to home, it could be a family member or significant other who cannot see the pain you are experiencing and sends the signal that you are making more of this pain than is necessary.

Level two: 0.7 to 2.3.   Your score is within the typical range for people who have chronic pain. You are moderately affected by the invisible nature of your pain and the lack of validation by others of your pain experience.

Level one: 0.6 or less.   A score at this level could mean that you have not felt invalidation of your pain experience. Alternatively, it could mean that you have worked through this experience and idea. This is good. Sometimes, people who score low on this scale tell me that they don't care what others think of them regarding their pain. These people have grown indifferent to what others think, and this may be working for them. Minimal endorsement of the ideas on this scale is a strength in your self-management of pain. You have likely been validated by others in your experience with chronic pain. Or perhaps your pain experience has been addressed by professionals, family, friends, and coworkers who have understood and accepted what you are going through. Finally, you may be the type of person who does not care what others think about your pain and your reaction to pain.

Invalidation and Pain

How important is it to feel validated and believed when you are living with pain? Apparently very important. How can a lack of validation affect your experience? For one thing, it taps your resources when they're already low just from dealing with chronic pain. There are days when you may think, *This hurts so bad I should be bleeding.* It just doesn't seem possible that anything you feel so intensely doesn't show. Many people say that sometimes they believe they have to prove to others they hurt, and this can frequently lead to behaviors like limping, bracing, or lying down. Increases in these behaviors can lead to increases in pain (as I'll explain in the next chapter), creating a vicious pain cycle.

Everyone would agree that wind is real. Just go outside on a windy day, and it cannot be denied. But we can't see the wind; we only see the effects of wind on other objects—the movement in the trees, the papers flying down the city street, kites in a park. Similarly, with pain, we often see the effects of pain in a person's behavior.

People sometimes tell me that they try to suppress the outward manifestations of their pain because they don't want the world to know about the pain. But then they are caught with the problem of feeling like the world doesn't understand them. One woman with whom I worked said she didn't want to be like her mother, who was a hypochondriac. So she hid her pain. But she has a nasty pain problem, and she is sincerely hurting. Her motivation is to not be a complainer, but she struggles greatly with hurting as much as she does. A man with whom I worked showed the opposite side of this coin. He wished others could feel or see his pain. He thought if he just had a crutch, a wheelchair, a neck brace, or a cast, the object would validate his pain without him having to say anything. Both of these people are not feeling validated, and both are suffering the psychological consequences of invalidation.

The feeling of invalidation of pain can set the stage for greater emotional suffering, mood problems, catastrophizing, and a sense of loss of control. When others do not believe that your pain is real, it is as if they are denying the wind to a person in the middle of a hurricane. For many people, lack of validation is a consequence of the invisible nature of pain. Whether or not people say it (and they sometimes do), what you hear is "You can't be in as much pain as you say you are." There is no obvious evidence of your pain. (It's not as if you turn green when you hurt.) Some people may question your sincerity and honesty and think you are manipulative. Others may question the authenticity of your pain and your pain complaints. You may begin to feel that your credibility and trustworthiness is being evaluated, and in fact, it likely is. Who wants to be accused of being manipulative, insincere, or untrustworthy?

You may begin to feel that no one believes you. Suspicion and paranoia are common reactions to chronic pain. These feelings may develop as time goes on and people become less solicitous. Or you may have just one person imply disbelief that your pain is as bad as you say it is, perhaps with a comment as innocent as "You look so strong. You don't look like you're in pain at all." Your suspicion that no one believes you can be even worse if you don't have a concrete diagnosis for your pain.

Medical Personnel and Invalidation of Pain

Sometimes seeking medical intervention will help your validation problems, especially if you get a concrete diagnosis. But sometimes medical personnel unwittingly make the problem worse. Perhaps you have felt frustrated when health care providers could not figure out what was causing your pain. You may even feel that you are letting your doctors down by not getting any better.

When your pain is not validated by health care professionals, you may begin to feel like a failure. You may wonder what's wrong with you that you are not getting better with all the help you are getting. You may start to wonder if your pain isn't real, if it's all in your head, if you're a hypochondriac, if you're a wimp. None of these are helpful thoughts.

Here are some more common, but unhelpful, thoughts related to a sense of invalidation by health care providers:

If my doctors could see my pain, maybe they would begin to realize what I have been worried about for so long and finally find the right treatment for me.

If my doctors could just see how bad my pain is, maybe they would stop blaming me for not getting better.

All I get are quick fixes that don't work: another pill or more physical therapy. When they see that all of this does not work, maybe they will finally appreciate what I have been saying.

Getting Better

Some people tell me that when they start to regain some function and feel better emotionally, they begin to doubt themselves and ask if getting better actually meant they did not have as much physical pain as they had thought. It is an interesting question that perhaps speaks more to a lack of appreciation of the biopsychosocial model than anything else. Pain is an intricate interaction of all three spheres, and improvement in one area does not imply that the other two did not play a role.

Dealing with Social Disbelief

Here are some tips for handling social disbelief and feelings of invalidation.

Get to know your medical condition. Regain control by mastering the medical jargon of your problem. You can begin by memorizing the names of muscles and nerves involved in your pain. Learn to pronounce the names of your medications. Words and knowledge can give you a sense of validity and control over your situation.

It may be helpful to look back into your past and ask yourself how pain was handled in your family of origin. What did your parents, siblings, or relatives do when they were in pain or had an accident? How did others react? Was there an indifference to pain, or would a pain problem or accident be a medical emergency for your family? Did you have any family members or relatives who had a chronic illness or pain problem? Looking back at how pain was handled and viewed may provide useful information for you today.

If you feel unsupported or misunderstood by family members, telling them how you are feeling and explaining your experiences with pain may be empowering. If you feel that others think you are lazy or lack motivation, you could share with them how pain reduces energy levels and leads to fatigue (show them chapter 6).

Guard against overgeneralizing on your part by assuming that people who don't understand your pain don't care about you or your relationship.

Work at effective communication and assertiveness. Talk to people around you about your condition and let them know what is going on inside you, physically and emotionally. Ask for what you need. And ask others what they are feeling in regard to your pain. Get those communication lines open. This may feel uncomfortable at first, but it will get better.

PRACTICING NEW IDEAS ABOUT PAIN

When your attention becomes entirely consumed by your body sensations, your pain worsens. This can lead you to interpret all bodily sensations as pain. The solution is to reestablish the idea that not all sensations equal pain. Deliberately plan some sensations that compete with pain, such as massage, light touch, or tickling. *Transcutaneous electrical nerve stimulation*, or TENS, is a kind of therapy that helps relieve pain by using electrical currents to create a tingling sensation and interfere with the transmission of pain signals.

Simple ideas about pain can shape and forge your experience with chronic pain. Now, here's a list of productive ideas you can work on to replace any unproductive ones:

I know that this pain flare-up is only temporary.

This pain flare-up is a reminder that I could practice my relaxation skills.

If I pace myself better and take a break now, I can still do my chores and get back on my routine.

The Chronic Pain Care Workbook

I need to stretch and relax throughout the day and pace myself better.

As a distraction to this pain that's starting to flare up, I could listen to some music or watch a movie.

My pain is starting to increase, so it is teaching me I need to take some deep breaths and see if I am bracing myself.

Even when I am hurting, I can enjoy things, and I can appreciate those times when I am hurting less.

If this pain is my enemy, what do I need to learn to do to outfox it?

I can have this pain and still do what I need to do, even if I do it a little slower.

TO SUM UP

This was a long chapter with a lot of information. Take a minute to think about all you learned. Look at your scores from each of the scales. You may find that you do a little of each of the seven kinds of thinking, or perhaps you do one more than the others. Consider how your scores influence one another (looking at your Pain Scorecard will help). You can see how some of these unproductive ideas even filter into other areas of your life, like sleep, sex, energy, daily activities, mood, and especially your interactions with other people.

Here's a brief roundup of what you learned in this chapter:

■ The ideas you have about pain can influence the way you cope with pain.

■ The seven common ideas (catastrophizing, fear of reinjury, expectation of a cure, self-blame, entitlement and frustration, future despair, and social disbelief) are associated with poor pain control and emotional upset.

■ You can learn to modify your thinking, challenge unproductive ideas, and construct a new, more realistic alternative way of thinking.

■ Modifying the way you view pain and experimenting with new ideas about living with pain requires work and practice. The more you practice, the better you can get.

Seeking help with challenging your ideas is healthy and beneficial. If you find you need assistance, see Resources for ways to make contact with professionals who can help.

In chapter 9, we move away from the realm of the psychosocial and back into the realm of the body with an exploration of pain behaviors: the things you do that alert others that you are in pain.

CHAPTER 9

Pain Behaviors

Pain behaviors are the signs of pain that others can see. Prominent pain psychologist Wilbert Fordyce (1976) coined the term "pain behavior" to capture all those things people do when they are in pain. Grimacing, bracing, wincing, moaning, limping, guarding, tensing, using a cane, talking about pain, clenching the teeth, taking pain medications, favoring a limb, crying: anything that communicates to another that you are in pain is a pain behavior. But pain behaviors are more than just an outward manifestation of pain. They are a form of communication to others, and your pain behaviors can be influenced by what others do.

In this chapter, we will take a close look at your pain behaviors and the messages you send to others about your pain. We will also examine what others do when you are in pain and the potential impact of these reactions on you.

Let's start by pinpointing your personal pain behaviors and determining whether they are a problem for you.

EXERCISE 9.1: PAIN BEHAVIORS SCALE

Rate how often you do each of the following *when you are in pain.*

moan or wince

	not at all						very frequently	
	0	1	2	3	4	5	6	7

lie down

	not at all						very frequently	
	0	1	2	3	4	5	6	7

brace yourself when you sit

> not at all   very frequently
>
> 0   1   2   3   4   5   6   7

walk in a way that others could notice that you are in pain

> not at all   very frequently
>
> 0   1   2   3   4   5   6   7

cry

> not at all   very frequently
>
> 0   1   2   3   4   5   6   7

become irritable

> not at all   very frequently
>
> 0   1   2   3   4   5   6   7

talk to others about your pain

> not at all   very frequently
>
> 0   1   2   3   4   5   6   7

tell others to leave you alone

> not at all   very frequently
>
> 0   1   2   3   4   5   6   7

To score this survey, add up all the numbers you circled, then divide the result by 8. This is your pain behavior score. This number should be between 0 and 7. Place your score on the Pain Scorecard.

Interpreting Your Score

Level three: 4.3 or more.   You are exhibiting more pain behaviors than is typical among people with chronic pain. Your score suggests that whether you want to or not, you are sending a loud message to others that you are in pain. Many people who feel invalidated by others because of the invisibility of their pain score high on both the Social Disbelief Scale (which you took in chapter 8) and the Pain Behaviors Scale. They want the world to know they are in pain, and one way to do that is to let the world see it.

Level two: 3.0 to 4.2.   You are within the average range for people with chronic pain.

Level one: 2.9 or less.   This is a lower than average level of pain behaviors for people with chronic pain. This suggests you are keeping your pain to yourself. Others may not even be aware that you have a chronic pain problem. Engaging in minimal pain behaviors may be working well for you; you may prefer that others not react to your pain. However, some people who score low on this scale struggle with the fact that others do not believe their pain is as bad as they say it is. You may feel you are putting on a false face to others. It may be nice not getting a lot of questions about pain or a lot of attention for pain, but at the same time, you may feel that others don't understand or appreciate the pain you are experiencing.

PAIN BEHAVIORS ARE A FORM OF COMMUNICATION

Fundamentally, pain behaviors are a form of communication. Pain behaviors can be defined by the fact that they are noticed by others. Your behavior sends the message that you are in pain. Pain can be communicated verbally or nonverbally, but either way, these behaviors tend to do one of two things. They can draw people toward you, soliciting sympathy and assistance (which some people like and some people hate) or they can push people away (which some people like and some people hate). You may display pain behaviors of which you aren't even aware, but the message is still being sent.

It can be enlightening to learn how others perceive and react to your pain behaviors. How do other people know when you are in pain, and what do they do when they see you in pain?

EXERCISE 9.2: HOW OTHERS SEE YOUR PAIN BEHAVIORS

Ask your partner (or a person who knows you well) to answer the following questions:

How do you know when I am in pain? What things do I do that send the message that I am hurting?

What do you do or say when you see me in pain? How do you react to me when I am in pain?

Take some time to think about the feedback you get from your spouse, partner, or loved one. Are you surprised by what you learned? How do you feel about the extent to which you engage in pain behaviors? Do you think your pain behaviors are drawing people toward you or pushing them away? Is this what you want?

Pain behaviors may not be the most effective way to communicate what you feel and what you need. In the remainder of this chapter, we'll look at some of the negative consequences of pain behaviors. I'll suggest some ways to change your pain behaviors and communicate your needs more effectively.

Share with your loved ones the notion that they are very important to you in your pain self-management program and that you are trying to make some changes and need their help. By talking to the important people in your life about the concept of pain behaviors, you can begin to include them in your pain management goals.

WHY CHANGE YOUR PAIN BEHAVIORS?

A high pain behavior score (level two or three) can be linked to several problems. Here are some of the most common:

- Guarded movement and bracing can cause you to avoid activities and suffer physical deconditioning.

- Bracing, guarding, and limping can cause increased pain in other parts of the body.

- Others may avoid interacting with you, and as a consequence, you may become isolated and depressed.

- Your needs and desires may be met, creating a negative feedback cycle in which you engage in more pain behaviors and further perpetuate your pain problem.

My research and that of others has shown that people who engage in a lot of pain behaviors also have significant problems with mood (including depression and anxiety) as well as sleep disturbances and difficulty with daily activities. So, as you can see, pain behaviors can have physical, psychological, and social consequences. Working to change pain behaviors is an important part of your pain self-management program since these behaviors affect so many other aspects of your life.

Let's take a closer look at the social conditioning loops that can develop with pain behaviors. It is the attention, or lack of attention, that is paid to your pain behaviors that matters. In many cases, pain behaviors solicit attention and support from others, which can often reinforce the behavior and create more pain behaviors.

For example, your spouse or partner may respond to you when you are in pain by giving you attention or by taking over your responsibilities. Essentially, you are rewarded for engaging in pain behaviors. Not surprisingly, this may ultimately elicit an increase in your pain behaviors. In this way, your pain behaviors may be shaped by your loved ones' reactions. People's expressions of pain increase if they experience positive consequences (such as attention or financial gains) or are able to avoid undesirable activities (such as work, chores, or stressful interactions with others) based on their displays of pain behaviors.

Avoiding chores may sound appealing at times, but don't forget the physical consequences of pain behaviors: physical deconditioning and strain on other parts of the body. Your goal is to experience less pain, not more.

YOU ARE MORE THAN YOUR PAIN BEHAVIORS

Many people with whom I work tell me that they do not want others to think that they have become their pain. They don't want to be defined by what is wrong with them. They want to show others that they are still who they used to be, not simply a chronic pain patient.

■ Bonnie

Bonnie was a fifty-six-year-old woman who had been diagnosed with fibromyalgia six years ago. She had retired early because the fibromyalgia made it difficult for her to work. She told me that she hated it when she ran into people she hadn't seen in a while and they asked her how her pain was. For a time, she had been open and honest with everyone who asked her about her pain, but this became overwhelming. She understood and appreciated their concern, but she wished people would talk about the old times or ask her about what she was doing now. So to avoid being defined by her pain, she put on a false face and said everything was fine. She hated the lie, but she hated the sympathy even more.

Bonnie's life changed when she decided to choose one person with whom she would talk openly about her pain. With one confidante, she was able to vent her feelings and be authentic about her pain experience without changing how everyone else saw her. She gained a sense of control with her pain experience that had been sorely lacking.

GETTING OTHERS TO TALK ABOUT SOMETHING BESIDES YOUR PAIN

Your pain may be a big part of your life. It may be the overriding subject on your mind. But you may not want to talk about it. You may want others to focus more on who you are than on how you feel. You may want them to be impressed with your accomplishments, not your illness. Whatever the reason, if you don't want to talk about your pain with everyone you meet every time you meet, be honest and tell others what you need. Communicate.

Try simply giving others permission to talk to you about other things besides your pain. You'll likely find people are relieved, not because they are bored or irritated by the subject (which you may fear), but rather because they want to help you but don't know how. By telling them straight up, you allow them to feel useful. They can then see you as a dynamic, complete, whole person. You may also find that people lighten up around you. Many people who don't know much about pain or illness are uncomfortable with people who aren't well because they aren't sure how they're supposed to treat people with pain. Don't be afraid to give them a road map and ease their discomfort.

▦ *Dennis*

Dennis was twenty-eight and had been diagnosed about a year earlier with complex regional pain syndrome, a chronic condition in which pain develops following a soft tissue injury or immobilization of an arm or leg. His pain had started with a twisted ankle about fourteen months prior, and continued with constant burning and intense pain. Many of Dennis's friends could not understand how a simple ankle sprain could lead to such long-term problems.

Dennis was understandably very frustrated with the pain, and he could see that his friends didn't know what to say or do for him. As a way of helping Dennis help his friends, I worked with him on a script he could use with his friends. Dennis came up with this:

> *I appreciate your concern about my pain and how I am doing, but I want to ask you a favor. I want you to not ask me about my pain anymore. It's always there anyway, so instead, please help me focus on other things. I will know that you care about me when you do this, and I will appreciate it. Thanks.*

In no time, not only did Dennis's friends stop asking him about his pain, but they also started coming around more and asking him to do more with them. Suddenly, his friends were less uncomfortable. They didn't know how to talk about chronic pain. Having permission to not do so freed them to talk about everything else.

Good communication can be an empowering replacement for pain behaviors. Learning to relax and becoming more aware of your body can also be powerful antidotes to pain behaviors.

RELAXATION AND BODY AWARENESS

You can modify pain behaviors such as limping, grimacing, bracing, and poor posture simply by becoming more aware of them. I was once told by my dentist that my teeth should be touching only when I was eating; the rest of the time, my teeth should be separated in a relaxed position. I began to notice that my teeth were frequently clenched during the day—my way of holding stress. With this new awareness (and the threat of dental surgery), I learned to relax my jaw and decrease my facial pain.

Try being more aware of your pain behaviors. Maybe even write them down for a few days or a week or more. Just being aware will modify the behavior.

The mirror in your bathroom or bedroom is your friend. Whenever you think of it, check your posture in the mirror. Are your shoulders level and even? Do you notice any correlation between your pain and your posture or the way you are holding yourself?

Consider videotaping yourself to see how you walk across a room, how you stand and sit, and even how you get out of a chair. Feedback can help facilitate change. Take time to focus on improving your posture and body movement, and see if it changes your pain experience.

Remember that belly breathing is a major relaxation strategy that helps combat muscle tension and fatigue, conditions that can increase pain behaviors. Take your blue dots (from exercise 6.2) and put them in places where you often feel stress (for example, on your telephone). Use them to remind you about good posture (in this case, not using your shoulder to hold the phone to your ear).

You may find it helpful to seek professional assistance with pain behaviors. This could include consultation with a physical therapist, an occupational therapist, or a biofeedback therapist (see Resources).

TO SUM UP

In this chapter, we have looked at how others see your pain through pain behaviors. We've discussed what pain behaviors are and how they affect you. We've talked about how you can get others to talk about something besides your pain, and you've learned to use relaxation and body awareness to gain control over your pain behaviors. You should now have a much better understanding of the messages you send with your behavior and how those messages are affecting your life.

In chapter 10, we will look at how pain changes your activity levels. You will learn how your thoughts can interfere with your activities and then discover what activities are most affected by your current circumstances.

CHAPTER 10

Activity Interference and Activity Avoidance

Pain changes your life. Typically, people simply do much less when they have chronic pain. In our culture, there is a pervasive belief that we are what we do. So if you have chronic pain and are doing less, who are you? Who and what do you become when you have a chronic pain problem? This chapter will help you answer these questions and more.

One of the complaints I hear most often concerning chronic pain is the difference between life before pain and life with pain. One of the more obvious changes is a radical drop in physical activity. Oftentimes this is due to physical limitations or limitations directly related to pain. But sometimes it has little to do with biology and everything to do with psychology. We need to consider both.

Activity interference describes the difference between the level of activity before the onset of your pain and your current activity level. Activity interference is part of the biological consequences of chronic pain. Many people in pain are simply no longer able to ride a bike, go camping, move the furniture to vacuum, or sometimes even go to work. Pain has interfered with their abilities to live the way they want.

Activity avoidance captures the psychological experience. It is more the anticipation of negative things to come. Activity avoidance is usually an emotional, psychological, and behavioral experience. It comes from the voice within you saying, *No, don't do that; it will hurt*. It's understandable to avoid activity if you expect it to cause pain. But problems arise when anticipation of pain and avoidance of activities stops you from experiencing life, ultimately causing your world to shrink.

The important distinction between interference and avoidance is that not all activity interference is directly related to having chronic pain. Other things can explain a change in activities besides pain. Activity avoidance is frequently related to fear and anxiety. It is valuable to know the difference between interference and avoidance, so the exercises in this chapter will help you evaluate both.

Our treatment goals will be to decrease activity avoidance and thus reduce activity interference due to pain.

EVALUATING YOUR ACTIVITY INTERFERENCE AND ACTIVITY AVOIDANCE

Let's take a look at how your activity levels have changed living with chronic pain. The exercises that follow ask how frequently you did these various activities of daily living prior to developing pain, how often you do them now, and how often you avoid them because of pain. The activities are broken down into five groups, including domestic activities, physically demanding activities, social activities, personal care activities (such as eating, walking, sleeping, and sex), and personal hygiene activities.

EXERCISE 10.1: INTERFERENCE AND AVOIDANCE SCALE FOR DOMESTIC ACTIVITIES

	How frequently did you do this activity *before* you had pain?	How frequently do you do this activity *now*?	Do you *avoid* this activity *because of pain*?
	not at all very often	not at all very often	not at all very often
running errands	0 1 2 3 4 5 6 7	0 1 2 3 4 5 6 7	0 1 2 3 4 5 6 7
laundry	0 1 2 3 4 5 6 7	0 1 2 3 4 5 6 7	0 1 2 3 4 5 6 7
ironing clothes	0 1 2 3 4 5 6 7	0 1 2 3 4 5 6 7	0 1 2 3 4 5 6 7
dusting or wiping	0 1 2 3 4 5 6 7	0 1 2 3 4 5 6 7	0 1 2 3 4 5 6 7
shopping for groceries	0 1 2 3 4 5 6 7	0 1 2 3 4 5 6 7	0 1 2 3 4 5 6 7
doing the dishes	0 1 2 3 4 5 6 7	0 1 2 3 4 5 6 7	0 1 2 3 4 5 6 7
preparing meals	0 1 2 3 4 5 6 7	0 1 2 3 4 5 6 7	0 1 2 3 4 5 6 7
vacuuming	0 1 2 3 4 5 6 7	0 1 2 3 4 5 6 7	0 1 2 3 4 5 6 7
scrubbing the floor	0 1 2 3 4 5 6 7	0 1 2 3 4 5 6 7	0 1 2 3 4 5 6 7
	"Before" score:	"Now" score:	
	Interference score:		Avoidance score:

Put a star next to those activities that are most important to you and that you would most like to bring back into your life.

To calculate your "before" score, add up the numbers you circled in the first column, then divide by 9.

To calculate your "now" score, add up the numbers you circled in the second column, then divide by 9.

To calculate your interference score, subtract your "now" score from your "before" score. This number should be between 0 and 7.

To calculate your avoidance score, add up the numbers you circled in the last column, then divide by 9.

Use your interference and avoidance scores to fill out the corresponding section of your Pain Scorecard.

Interpreting Your Score

Let's look first at your activity interference score for domestic tasks. The average score for people with chronic pain is 1.1 to 2.6; a score in this range places you at level two on the Pain Scorecard. Level one is 1.0 or less. Level three is 2.7 or more. It's quite common for people with chronic pain to have difficulty with domestic activities. The average person with chronic pain does not engage in many of these household tasks once they develop the pain problem.

Keep in mind that men and women tend to score differently on the "before" measure, with women scoring higher. Of course, if you live alone, you may not have a choice of not doing some of these activities, regardless of your pain.

Now let's look at your avoidance score for domestic activities. The average score for people with chronic pain is 2.7 to 4.5; a score in this range places you at level two on the Pain Scorecard. Level one is 2.6 or less. Level three is 4.6 or more.

Take a close look at those individual activities that you rated 5, 6, or 7 in column three, and ask yourself if you want or need to engage in these activities in the future. If you do, then you could use this activity as a target behavior for modification and pacing exercises.

Take a moment to look at any activities that have not changed from before to now and make a note of them. Ask yourself if this unchanged activity is important to you, and ask why it hasn't changed. If the activity is important to you, it may be useful to remind yourself that you still do it, especially if you catastrophize about your pain and think that pain has stopped you from doing "everything." It obviously hasn't.

EXERCISE 10.2: REFLECT ON YOUR INTERFERENCE AND AVOIDANCE SCORES FOR DOMESTIC ACTIVITIES

Your scores on the Interference and Avoidance Scale for Domestic Activities raise some pretty important questions. Take a moment to answer the following so you can see how your household activities have changed since you developed chronic pain.

What activities have changed the least? Are they important activities to you?

What activities have changed or decreased the most? Are they important activities to you?

Is someone else picking up this task, or is it going undone?

What effect is it having on you if this activity is not happening?

What does this mean, and does it say anything about you?

What activities did you mark with a star to indicate that you want to bring them back into your life?

Now let's move on to the next category, physically demanding activities.

EXERCISE 10.3: INTERFERENCE AND AVOIDANCE SCALE FOR PHYSICALLY DEMANDING ACTIVITIES

	How frequently did you do this activity *before* you had pain?	How frequently do you do this activity *now*?	Do you *avoid* this activity *because of pain*?
	not at all very often	not at all very often	not at all very often
moving furniture	0 1 2 3 4 5 6 7	0 1 2 3 4 5 6 7	0 1 2 3 4 5 6 7
hunting/ fishing	0 1 2 3 4 5 6 7	0 1 2 3 4 5 6 7	0 1 2 3 4 5 6 7
mowing the lawn	0 1 2 3 4 5 6 7	0 1 2 3 4 5 6 7	0 1 2 3 4 5 6 7
working on the car	0 1 2 3 4 5 6 7	0 1 2 3 4 5 6 7	0 1 2 3 4 5 6 7
gardening	0 1 2 3 4 5 6 7	0 1 2 3 4 5 6 7	0 1 2 3 4 5 6 7
doing light household repairs	0 1 2 3 4 5 6 7	0 1 2 3 4 5 6 7	0 1 2 3 4 5 6 7
playing sports	0 1 2 3 4 5 6 7	0 1 2 3 4 5 6 7	0 1 2 3 4 5 6 7
washing the car	0 1 2 3 4 5 6 7	0 1 2 3 4 5 6 7	0 1 2 3 4 5 6 7
driving long distances	0 1 2 3 4 5 6 7	0 1 2 3 4 5 6 7	0 1 2 3 4 5 6 7
doing plumbing repair	0 1 2 3 4 5 6 7	0 1 2 3 4 5 6 7	0 1 2 3 4 5 6 7
	"Before" score:	"Now" score:	
	Interference score:		Avoidance score:

Put a star next to those activities that are most important to you and that you would most like to bring back into your life.

To calculate your "before" score, add up the numbers you circled in the first column, then divide by 10.

To calculate your "now" score, add up the numbers you circled in the second column, then divide by 10.

To calculate your interference score, subtract your "now" score from your "before" score. This number should be between 0 and 7.

To calculate your avoidance score, add up the numbers you circled in the last column, then divide by 10.

Use your interference and avoidance scores to fill out the corresponding section of your Pain Scorecard.

Interpreting Your Score

Let's look first at your activity interference score for physically demanding activities. The average score for people with chronic pain is 1.9 to 3.4; a score in this range places you at level two on the Pain Scorecard. Level one is 1.8 or less. Level three is 3.5 or more. A significant drop in physically demanding activities is typical for people who have chronic pain. You likely will not be moving heavy furniture with a chronic pain problem. Becoming aware of your physical capacities is a valuable lesson to learn from pain. For the most part, physically demanding activities should be reduced, modified, or even eliminated when you have a chronic pain condition. However, this is not to say that you should give up exercising. As you know by now, a carefully designed exercise program is a valuable tool in reducing pain.

Among people with chronic pain, the average avoidance score for physically demanding activities is between 3.5 and 5.5. A score at this level places you at level two on the Pain Scorecard. Level one is 3.4 or less; level three is 5.6 or more.

As you can see, most people in pain tend to avoid these heavy activities, and this may be very appropriate. Take a close look at those individual activities that you rated 5, 6, or 7 and ask yourself if you want or need to engage in these activities in the future. If you do, check with your physician or other health care providers to see if they endorse an increase in this activity. If so, you could use this activity as a target behavior for modification and pacing exercises.

EXERCISE 10.4: REFLECT ON YOUR INTERFERENCE AND AVOIDANCE SCORES FOR PHYSICALLY DEMANDING ACTIVITIES

Take a moment to answer the following questions so you can see how your participation in physically demanding activities has changed since you developed chronic pain.

What activities have changed the least? Are they important activities to you?

Which have changed the most? Are they important activities to you?

Is someone else picking up this activity, or is it going undone?

What effect is it having on you if this activity is not happening?

What does this mean, and does it say anything about you?

What activities did you mark with a star to indicate that you want to bring them back into your life?

Next, let's take a look at how chronic pain has affected your social life.

EXERCISE 10.5: INTERFERENCE AND AVOIDANCE SCALE FOR SOCIAL ACTIVITIES

	How frequently did you do this activity *before* you had pain?	How frequently do you do this activity *now*?	Do you *avoid* this activity *because of pain*?
	not at all very often	not at all very often	not at all very often
dining out	0 1 2 3 4 5 6 7	0 1 2 3 4 5 6 7	0 1 2 3 4 5 6 7
going to parties	0 1 2 3 4 5 6 7	0 1 2 3 4 5 6 7	0 1 2 3 4 5 6 7
going to a walk-in movie	0 1 2 3 4 5 6 7	0 1 2 3 4 5 6 7	0 1 2 3 4 5 6 7
going to nightclubs	0 1 2 3 4 5 6 7	0 1 2 3 4 5 6 7	0 1 2 3 4 5 6 7
dancing	0 1 2 3 4 5 6 7	0 1 2 3 4 5 6 7	0 1 2 3 4 5 6 7
being visited by others	0 1 2 3 4 5 6 7	0 1 2 3 4 5 6 7	0 1 2 3 4 5 6 7
	"Before" score:	"Now" score:	
	Interference score:		Avoidance score:

Put a star next to those activities that are most important to you and that you would most like to bring back into your life.

To calculate your "before" score, add up the numbers you circled in the first column, then divide by 6.

To calculate your "now" score, add up the numbers you circled in the second column, then divide by 6.

To calculate your interference score, subtract your "now" score from your "before" score. This number should be between 0 and 7.

To calculate your avoidance score, add up the numbers you circled in the last column, then divide by 6.

Use your interference and avoidance scores to fill out the corresponding section of your Pain Scorecard.

Interpreting Your Score

It has been my clinical experience that high social activity interference scores are associated with mood-related problems such as depression. An interference score of 2.4 or higher places you in level three, 0.7 to 2.3 is level two, and 0.6 or less is level one. Avoidance of social activities can also place you at risk for mood problems. Among people with chronic pain, the average avoidance score for social activities is between 2.5 and 4.5. This places you at level two on the Pain Scorecard. Scores of 2.4 or less are level one; scores of 4.6 or more are level three.

In this scale, it's worthwhile to consider your "before" score. If your "before" score was more than 3.9, you used to engage in more social activities than the average person who later developed chronic pain. You may be especially vulnerable to mood-related problems if your social activities drop off significantly and you become isolated. On the other hand, if your "before" score was less than 2.4, you engaged in less socializing than the typical person who later developed chronic pain. A low "before" score suggests that you may not believe social activities are very important. This may just be your style, and there is nothing wrong with this.

Depression and isolation can significantly amplify your experience of chronic pain. When you're setting goals in your self-management program, you'll want to pay special attention to maintaining or increasing social activities and regaining your connections with other people. This is especially important if you were a very social person before you developed chronic pain.

EXERCISE 10.6: REFLECT ON YOUR INTERFERENCE AND AVOIDANCE SCORES FOR SOCIAL ACTIVITIES

Take a moment to answer the following questions so you can see how your social activities have changed since the development of chronic pain.

Which of your social activities have changed the least? Are they important activities to you?

Which have changed or decreased the most? Are they important activities to you?

What effect is it having on you that you aren't engaging in this activity?

What does this mean, and does it say anything about you?

What activities did you mark with a star to indicate that you want to bring them back into your life?

Let's look at how chronic pain has affected your participation in personal care activities.

EXERCISE 10.7: INTERFERENCE AND AVOIDANCE SCALE FOR PERSONAL CARE ACTIVITIES

	How frequently did you do this activity *before* you had pain?	How frequently do you do this activity *now*?	Do you *avoid* this activity *because of pain*?
	not at all very often	not at all very often	not at all very often
eating	0 1 2 3 4 5 6 7	0 1 2 3 4 5 6 7	0 1 2 3 4 5 6 7
walking long distances	0 1 2 3 4 5 6 7	0 1 2 3 4 5 6 7	0 1 2 3 4 5 6 7
sleeping	0 1 2 3 4 5 6 7	0 1 2 3 4 5 6 7	0 1 2 3 4 5 6 7
sexual activity	0 1 2 3 4 5 6 7	0 1 2 3 4 5 6 7	0 1 2 3 4 5 6 7
	"Before" score:	"Now" score:	
	Interference score:		Avoidance score:

Put a star next to those activities that are most important to you and that you would most like to bring back into your life.

To calculate your "before" score, add up the numbers you circled in the first column, then divide by 4.

To calculate your "now" score, add up the numbers you circled in the second column, then divide by 4.

To calculate your interference score, subtract your "now" score from your "before" score. This number should be between 0 and 7.

To calculate your avoidance score, add up the numbers you circled in the last column, then divide by 4.

Use your interference and avoidance scores to fill out the corresponding section of your Pain Scorecard.

Interpreting Your Score

An interference score of 2.6 or higher places you in level three, 1.2 to 2.5 is level two, and 1.1 or less is level one. Among people with chronic pain, the average avoidance score for personal care activities is 2.4 to 4.0. A score in this range places you at level two. Level one is 2.3 or less; level three is 4.1 or more.

This activity category encompasses critical life functioning behaviors: sleep, which has a tremendous impact on energy and fatigue; eating, which is the foundation of nutrition; walking, which is fundamental to movement; and sexual activity. If chronic pain is significantly interfering with these activities, or if you're avoiding these activities because of pain, you'll need to prioritize working on this area. Chapter 6 includes detailed suggestions about sleep, movement, and nutrition. I'll discuss sex in chapter 13.

EXERCISE 10.8: REFLECT ON YOUR INTERFERENCE AND AVOIDANCE SCORES FOR PERSONAL CARE ACTIVITIES

Take a moment to answer the following questions so you can see how chronic pain has affected your personal care activities.

Which of these activities have changed the least? How important are these activities to you?

Which activities have changed or decreased the most? How important are these activities to you?

What effect is it having on you if this activity is not happening?

What does this mean, and does it say anything about you?

What activities did you mark with a star to indicate that you want to bring them back into your life?

Finally, let's take a look at how chronic pain has affected your personal hygiene activities.

EXERCISE 10.9: INTERFERENCE AND AVOIDANCE SCALE FOR PERSONAL HYGIENE ACTIVITIES

	How frequently did you do this activity *before* you had pain? not at all very often	How frequently do you do this activity *now*? not at all very often	Do you *avoid* this activity *because of pain*? not at all very often
getting dressed	0 1 2 3 4 5 6 7	0 1 2 3 4 5 6 7	0 1 2 3 4 5 6 7
brushing or combing your hair	0 1 2 3 4 5 6 7	0 1 2 3 4 5 6 7	0 1 2 3 4 5 6 7
showering	0 1 2 3 4 5 6 7	0 1 2 3 4 5 6 7	0 1 2 3 4 5 6 7
brushing your teeth	0 1 2 3 4 5 6 7	0 1 2 3 4 5 6 7	0 1 2 3 4 5 6 7
shaving	0 1 2 3 4 5 6 7	0 1 2 3 4 5 6 7	0 1 2 3 4 5 6 7
	"Before" score:	"Now" score:	
	Interference score:		Avoidance score:

Put a star next to those activities that are most important to you and that you would most like to bring back into your life.

To calculate your "before" score, add up the numbers you circled in the first column, then divide by 5.

To calculate your "now" score, add up the numbers you circled in the second column, then divide by 5.

To calculate your interference score, subtract your "now" score from your "before" score. This number should be between 0 and 7.

To calculate your avoidance score, add up the numbers you circled in the last column, then divide by 5.

Use your interference and avoidance scores to fill out the corresponding section of your Pain Scorecard.

Interpreting Your Score

An interference score of 0.9 or higher places you in level three, 0.2 to 0.8 is level two, and 0.1 or less is level one. Among people with chronic pain, the average avoidance score for personal hygiene activities is 0.7 to 2.3. A score in this range places you at level two. Level one is 0.6 or less; level three is 2.4 or more.

The location of your pain will influence your scores on this scale. If your pain is primarily in your neck, head, shoulder, or arm, you will show greater changes on this scale than a person who has back, leg, or foot pain. This makes sense, since several of the activities (such as shaving and combing your hair) require raising your arms and hands above the shoulders.

EXERCISE 10.10: REFLECT ON YOUR INTERFERENCE AND AVOIDANCE SCORES FOR PERSONAL HYGIENE ACTIVITIES

Take a moment to answer the following questions so you can see how chronic pain has affected your personal hygiene activities.

Which personal hygiene activities have changed the least? How important are these activities to you?

What activities have changed or decreased the most? Are they important activities to you?

What effect is it having on you if this activity is not happening?

What does this mean, and does it say anything about you?

What activities did you mark with a star to indicate that you want to bring them back into your life?

Your activity interference and avoidance scores show you what activities have been most affected by your pain experience. The higher the scores, the greater the impact on your life. Use the Pain Score-card to see your scores for all five categories at a glance. Whether you've lost activities through interference or avoidance, gaining back some of the activities of living is an important goal in your pain self-management program.

Here are some suggestions to focus your resources and direct your attention where it will do the most good. First, determine how important each activity category is in your life. One way to do this is to look at how many activities you starred and in what categories. These activities can become your treatment goals for the exercises in the next part of this chapter and throughout the book. Later in this chapter, you will learn how to break these activities down into small and meaningful steps and how to modify them in ways that keep them in your life. Second, determine which activities are physically counterproductive and possibly damaging or dangerous. For example, your physician may have recommended that you not engage in heavy lifting or certain other strenuous activities. You may simply have to give up some activities. Other tasks can be done by someone else in your household or by a paid helper.

OVERCOMING ACTIVITY INTERFERENCE

But what about the things you really miss, like playing basketball with your kids or going to a restaurant with friends? Now that you've identified the activities that are most important to you, let's take a look at how you can claim your life back from chronic pain. In this section, we'll explore three options: first, using goal setting, pacing, and activity quotas to resume activities; second, modifying activities you can still do, but not the way you used to; and third, exploring alternatives to activities that are important to you but that you simply can no longer do safely.

Unlearning "The More I Do, the More I Hurt"

Here's a scenario that is all too familiar. While conducting my initial evaluations, I ask people how active they were before their pain problem began, and they tell me that they used to be very active. They used to ski, hike, camp, fish, go to the movies, ride motorcycles, and so on. But because of their pain problems, they have stopped all of those activities and are not doing much at all beyond resting and lying down—all due to pain. They tell me that pain has stopped them from doing "everything" they used to do. They tell me that they have come to learn that the more they do, the more they hurt.

Frequently, people with chronic pain come to the conclusion that their level of activity is directly related to the severity of their pain. They push themselves until they feel the pain, and then the pain tells them to stop. They rest until they feel the pain ease, and then they repeat the same pattern again and again. Think back to the discussion of elevators and escalators in chapter 6. The elevator scenario—overactivity followed by inactivity—is a vicious cycle that leads to frustration and despair, physical deconditioning, muscle weakness, fatigue, sleep problems, isolation, and depression. Pain begins to take control of your life, and you feel helpless.

Pacing

When you're on the elevator, every time you are active, your pain flares up. You learn that increased activity is paired with increased pain. In reality, this isn't a problem of too much activity; it is a problem of too little pacing. Pacing is the key to breaking the paired association between "the more I do" and "the more I hurt." The pattern of overdoing and underdoing is dangerous. It is the major reason people end up inadvertently perpetuating their pain problems. You can become your own worst enemy. I want to help you establish a new set of skills and behaviors that will help you regain control of your life.

Using Activity Quotas

One proven way to increase activity levels gradually and safely is through *activity quotas*, a system originally developed by Wilbert Fordyce (1976). In this system, just as you would expect, physical activity—prescribed systematically in gradually increasing amounts—is rewarded with rest. So, rather than allowing your pain level to determine your activity level, you engage in predetermined safe and tolerable levels of activity. Such activity is followed by a planned, rather than pain-contingent, period of rest. The aim is to arrange things so you increase activities with the least amount of pain.

Goal Setting

Start by choosing a goal. Review the exercises you completed earlier in this chapter, and consider which activities you would most like to resume. Depending on your goal and your level of pain, you may want to talk with your doctor or physical therapist. Once you have a goal in mind, you can develop an activity quota plan.

For example, suppose you really want to attend your daughter's graduation from college in six months. You're concerned because walking is painful for you and you get out of breath easily. You know that on the day of the event, you will need to get from the campus entrance to the amphitheater, and you'd like to be able to walk there without help. You make an appointment with your doctor, who gives you the go-ahead for a very gentle exercise program. With your doctor's approval, you begin by walking slowly each day for five minutes without stopping, then resting for twenty minutes. After two weeks of this, you increase to walking ten minutes, still resting afterward. After four more weeks, you walk for fifteen minutes at a time, and you pick up the pace a bit. Even though you usually feel pretty good, you resist the temptation to walk farther or skip resting. You continue to incrementally increase your distance and your pace, and by the time graduation rolls around, you feel confident that you'll be able to get where you need to go and enjoy the day.

This exercise will help you reach your objective by choosing a realistic goal and pacing yourself properly.

EXERCISE 10.11: CHOOSE A REALISTIC GOAL AND PACE YOURSELF

Start by choosing a goal that is realistic, meaningful, achievable, and specific. Remember that your goal doesn't need to be to get back to your old life. Instead, find a goal that engages you more in the life possible now. Write it down.

My goal is:

To begin, I will _____ (activity) for _____ (length of time), then rest for _____ (length of time). I will do this _____ (frequency).

After _____ (number) weeks, I will _____ (activity) for _____ (length of time), then rest for _____ (length of time). I will do this _____ (frequency).

After _____ (number) weeks, I will _____ (activity) for _____ (length of time), then rest for _____ (length of time). I will do this _____ (frequency).

Using Exercise to Reach Your Goals

Movement is going to be key to many of your goals about regaining activities, and exercise is the best way to increase your capacity for movement. Exercise can also help you overcome the idea that any activity beyond the minimal is damaging. Check with your doctor to be sure exercise is safe for you. A physical therapist can help you develop a graduated exercise program that takes into account your individual needs. Choose an activity that you like, and you will be much more likely to exercise regularly and enjoy the benefits. Beginning an exercise program usually leads to some discomfort, but keep in mind the distinction between normal soreness ("hurt") and damage ("harm").

Remember to pace yourself. If you have a tendency to overdo it, consider using a watch with an alarm or a kitchen timer to gently remind yourself that you need to stop and take a break.

The long-term benefits of exercise, such as increased muscle strength, flexibility, and sense of well-being, are all within your reach. For more discussion of exercise, see chapter 6.

Modifying Activities

Flexibility and adaptability play a major role in setting realistic and achievable goals. Your ability to modify past activities to meet the demands of your current life with chronic pain becomes a critical survival skill.

Instead of completely giving up the game of golf due to arthritis, Susan was able to modify her ideas about playing golf and was able to continue to enjoy her friends and the game of golf.

■ Susan

Susan was forty-five and suffered from arthritis. She loved golf. She said she was never very good, but the game made her happier than anything else in her life. She especially liked golfing with her girlfriends. After several years of frequent flare-ups of arthritis pain, she stopped playing golf and didn't see much of her friends. Just swinging the driver off the tee was enough to put her in bed for a week. She was unable to work because of her pain condition, and years of being on disability had depleted her finances. Not only was her pain interfering with her golf, she could no longer afford it. She was understandably angry and depressed.

What is important about Susan's story is that she was an all-or-nothing person and thought in terms of black and white. Either she would play an eighteen-hole round of golf, or she wouldn't play at all. My challenge with Susan was to address her all-or-nothing thinking and help her understand the role it was playing in her life. We started off by defining "playing golf." Initially, she defined "playing golf" as playing eighteen holes. I was able to persuade her to modify her thinking and expand her definition of "playing golf" to include simply practicing putting on the practice green for an hour. I asked Susan if she could practice putting (something that involves minimal effort with no large swing) without aggravating her pain, and she agreed. Her goal was to invite two of her girlfriends to join her on the practice putting green and "play golf" for about an hour.

The putting game allowed her to bring golf back into her life, increased her social interaction, and cost her nothing. Her fun meter went up along with her activity levels, and her level of depression went down—just like the putts she took on the putting green.

Exploring Alternatives

Sometimes, modifying activities is impossible due to your pain and your physical condition. Giving up certain activities can be difficult, but if you look at what that activity meant to you and the role it played in your life, you may begin to find some acceptable alternatives. For example, suppose you used to really enjoy playing basketball with your kids, but this is now out of the question for physical reasons. You realize that one of the most important things you got out of playing basketball with your kids was spending quality time with them and teaching them the game. You may find that acting as a volunteer assistant coach for their YMCA team could fulfill those needs without putting you at risk of a major pain flare-up.

OVERCOMING ACTIVITY AVOIDANCE

People experiencing chronic pain avoid many activities, but not always because of physical limitations. It may be that you steer clear of things you *think* will cause you pain.

Confronters and Avoiders

You have likely answered the avoidance questions in one of two possible ways: as a confronter or as an avoider. The higher your scores on the avoidance scales, the more likely you are an avoider. Check your Pain Scorecard to get an overall impression. If you consistently scored in levels two and three, you are an avoider, and you are not alone.

Avoiders tend to shy away from activities because of the anticipation of pain rather than as a direct response to pain. Avoidance of activities becomes the rule rather than the exception, and your world begins to shrink. This is because when you start to avoid a lot of activities due to pain, you have fewer opportunities to engage in activities and *not* experience pain. As a result, you conclude that activity causes pain, and you continue to avoid activity.

As you now know, both physical inactivity and social isolation may worsen your pain problem. Using an avoidance strategy to cope with pain can become an ingrained pattern that perpetuates your chronic pain. Furthermore, research suggests that people with acute pain who fear movement and avoid physical activities are more likely to eventually develop a chronic pain problem (Philips 1988; Vlaeyen and Linton 2000). Pain-related fear, attention to pain, and activity avoidance apparently play a major role in keeping pain going and making it worse.

As you can see, activity avoidance rests on the same "The more I do, the more I hurt" belief that underlies activity interference. The solution is the same: slow, steady, gradual increases in activities without the paired association of increases in pain. When you take the escalator approach to activity, you get several pain management benefits. Your emotional reactions (depression, anxiety, and anger) diminish, you recognize that pain varies in different situations and circumstances, and you learn that high pain level is not always linked to increased activity. In exercise 10.11, you learned how to use goal setting and pacing to break the association between "the more I do" and "the more I hurt." You also learned in chapter 8 that you can modify your ideas about living with pain—specifically, fears of reinjury and the idea that hurt means harm. Since activity avoidance is largely a problem of ideas or beliefs, you might find it helpful to use the Thought Evaluation Form (exercise 8.2).

If your activity avoidance scores are primarily in level one, you can be considered a confronter. Confronters generally view pain as something temporary and are prepared to face the pain. In a sense, not avoiding activities may be a form of acceptance of pain and an example of engaging in life despite having pain. Reducing avoidance and gradually increasing your exposure to activity and potential pain can lead to a psychological sense of increased control. If you are a confronter, mood-related problems and other psychosocial problems may likely be of minor concern.

TO SUM UP

You now know that pairing "the more I do" with "the more I hurt" is a bad idea. This pairing will keep you from moving, and movement is life. Although it is not the only negative pain cycle, it is one of the most destructive.

Activity avoidance and activity interference change your daily life. This chapter focused on how the elements of your daily life have been affected by your pain experience and encouraged you to take a close look at what you may need to do differently.

Chapter 11 will present the "other" pain that most people in chronic pain experience—that is, emotional pain and suffering. Living with chronic pain taxes the system and exacts a cost. That cost is emotional. It can take the form of depression, worry, anxiety, anger, and diminished quality of life. In the next chapter, we will take a look at the emotional price you are paying living with chronic pain.

CHAPTER 11

Emotional Pain and Suffering

Chronic pain and mood problems go together. As it gets harder and harder to cope, as the pain limits your participation in pleasurable activities, mood-related problems such as depression, anxiety, and anger can set in. Addressing and treating mood-related problems allows you to more fully engage in other aspects of your pain self-management program. In this chapter, we will take a close look at depression, anger, and anxiety—and humor—as they relate to your pain experience.

Negative emotions are not simply undesired side effects of pain. They can be powerful determinants of your pain experience. But it's not all bad. There may be some benefit to unsettled emotions. Negative emotions increase your attention to the threat of tissue damage and promote recovery by leading you to avoid those things that could make your pain worse. Also, negative emotions such as anger and anxiety could be viewed as important in helping you escape or deal with external threats other than pain. Pain-increasing responses such as hypervigilance, muscle tension, and agitation play an important role in enabling an effective and quick response in the face of *acute* pain. However, in the face of chronic pain, these mechanisms may no longer be helpful.

Over the long term, depression, anxiety, and anger focus your mind on pain and sensitize both the body and the mind to pain. For most people, these emotions cause ongoing stress, tension, and frustration, which creates a greater sensitivity to your pain signals. Plus, continually trying to escape or avoid pain can increase your level of pain. Simply put, depression, anxiety, and anger can make chronic pain worse.

DEPRESSION

Studies have shown that 30 percent to 65 percent of people experiencing chronic pain are or will become depressed (Sullivan et al. 1992). Compare this to the 5 percent to 17 percent of the general population who are or will be depressed (Kessler et al. 2003), and you start to see the extent of the problem.

Chronic pain can lead to decreased activity, reduced self-esteem, a sense of despondency and hopelessness, and a decreased sense of control over pain. Reducing depression as part of your pain self-management program may actually help increase your physical activity, and by now, you know how important this is.

The sensation of pain can bring you further into yourself and focus your attention on any and all body sensations and thoughts. Sight, sound, taste, touch, and smell all help you explore the world outside yourself. They tend to take you out of yourself and focus you on the world around you.

Let's take a look at where your attention is focused, especially when you start to experience a pain flare-up.

EXERCISE 11.1: ANTICIPATED EMOTIONAL DISTRESS SCALE

When your pain increases sharply, how concerned are you that

you will become angry

	not at all concerned					very concerned	
0	1	2	3	4	5	6	7

you will become irritable

	not at all concerned					very concerned	
0	1	2	3	4	5	6	7

you will "lose your mind"

	not at all concerned					very concerned	
0	1	2	3	4	5	6	7

you will have a nervous breakdown

	not at all concerned					very concerned	
0	1	2	3	4	5	6	7

you will become increasingly dependent upon others

	not at all concerned					very concerned	
0	1	2	3	4	5	6	7

you will become depressed

	not at all concerned					very concerned	
0	1	2	3	4	5	6	7

you will lose self-respect

	not at all concerned					very concerned	
0	1	2	3	4	5	6	7

To score this exercise, add up all the numbers you circled, then divide by 7. This is your anticipated emotional distress score. This number should be between 0 and 7. Place your score in your Pain Scorecard.

Interpreting Your Score

The higher your score, the more you are concerned about potential emotional suffering related to your pain and future pain flare-ups. The opposite is true with lower scores.

Level three: 3.4 or more. You worry significantly that your quality of life will suffer and that future pain flare-ups will ruin your emotional well-being and self-esteem. Anticipated emotional distress is a major area of concern in your pain self-management program.

Level two: 1.5 to 3.3. Your score indicates a level of concern with the emotional impact of future pain flare-ups comparable to that experienced by most people with chronic pain. Anticipated emotional distress is an area of concern for your self-management program. You could benefit from some of the treatment suggestions in this chapter.

Level one: 1.4 or less. You are anticipating minimal future emotional distress related to pain flare-ups. Chances are your scores on the other depression and anxiety scales will also show minimal problems. Consider this a major asset in your pain self-management program.

If you scored at level two or three, the stage is set for you to also score high on the scales that measure depression, anxiety, and entitlement/frustration. You are likely suffering emotionally from your current chronic pain experience and anticipation of future pain flare-ups.

Let's evaluate whether you're currently experiencing symptoms of depression.

EXERCISE 11.2: DEPRESSION SCALE

Over the past two weeks, how often have you experienced the following symptoms?

crying easily

not at all						very often	
0	1	2	3	4	5	6	7

feelings of guilt

not at all						very often	
0	1	2	3	4	5	6	7

worrying

	not at all						very often
0	1	2	3	4	5	6	7

disappointment in yourself

	not at all						very often
0	1	2	3	4	5	6	7

feelings of anger

	not at all						very often
0	1	2	3	4	5	6	7

feelings of sadness or depression

	not at all						very often
0	1	2	3	4	5	6	7

feelings of worthlessness

	not at all						very often
0	1	2	3	4	5	6	7

feelings of inferiority

	not at all						very often
0	1	2	3	4	5	6	7

decreased interest in socializing

	not at all						very often
0	1	2	3	4	5	6	7

loss of interest for a variety of previously pleasant activities

	not at all						very often
0	1	2	3	4	5	6	7

thoughts of harming yourself or "ending it all"

	not at all						very often
0	1	2	3	4	5	6	7

being discouraged about the future

	not at all						very often
0	1	2	3	4	5	6	7

feelings of being punished or deserving punishment

      not at all   very often

        0   1   2   3   4   5   6   7

difficulty motivating yourself to do things

      not at all   very often

        0   1   2   3   4   5   6   7

To score this exercise, add up all the numbers you circled, then divide by 14. This is your depression score. This number should be between 0 and 7. Place your score in your Pain Scorecard.

Interpreting Your Score

Your depression score is a reflection of the emotional toll that pain has taken on your life.

Level three: 3.4 or more.   Depression has become a major part of your chronic pain experience, and it will be a major area of concern in managing your pain experience. Remember that many people with chronic pain become depressed. You are not weak or crazy for experiencing symptoms of depression. Your pain self-management program must include addressing the emotional suffering you are experiencing. It's important that you take your depression as seriously as your chronic pain problem. You would almost certainly benefit from consulting a mental health professional about your depression (see Resources for information about finding providers in your area). The good news is that depression can be treated effectively, and with effective treatment of depression, you will likely see an improvement in your chronic pain problem.

According to my research, people who have high depression scores, high pain behavior scores, and high activity interference scores tend to be particularly distressed and dysfunctional. If you scored high in all three areas, you are much more likely to be coping poorly with your pain problem.

Level two: 1.7 to 3.3.   Your score is within the typical range for people who have chronic pain. However, an average or typical score is still high compared to the average person who does not have chronic pain. A score at level two indicates that you are moderately burdened by depression and could use assistance with depression management.

Level one: 1.6 or less.   You have minimal difficulty with depressive symptoms. This is not an area of particular concern in your pain self-management program.

Depression and Self-Esteem

Taking a closer look at the items that make up this scale can give you insight into effective treatment strategies. Look at the numbers you circled for "disappointment in yourself," "feelings of worthlessness," and "feelings of inferiority." These items tap into self-esteem: how you feel about yourself. If you scored relatively high on these items, it's likely that pain is magnifying these feelings and affecting the core of who you are.

If chronic pain is damaging your self-esteem, consider these treatment recommendations:

■ Set realistic and achievable goals to give yourself a sense of accomplishment.

■ Avoid discounting the positive when good things happen in your life; accept affirmations from others.

■ Remember that you are more than your pain.

■ Develop coping statements that affirm your worth separate from your identity as a person with chronic pain.

■ Modify activities you previously enjoyed so that you can do those things successfully (see chapter 10 for suggestions about activity modification).

■ Examine any unproductive ideas you have about living with chronic pain (see chapter 8).

Chronic pain often decreases your ability to engage in activities that used to be fun and pleasurable. Take a look at your activity interference scores (from the exercises in chapter 10) and see how many previously pleasant activities are now limited by pain. All of these difficulties can add to a loss of self-esteem.

Depression and Other Experiences and Thoughts About Pain

Research studies have shown that the intensity of pain, the frequency of severe pain episodes, and the number of painful areas of the body are significant predictors of the development of depression in people who have chronic pain (Nicassio and Wallston 1992).

> *People who have something better to do don't hurt as much.*
>
> —Wilbert Fordyce

My research has shown that depression correlates highly with sleep disturbance, catastrophizing about pain, self-blame, and avoidance of socializing. Check your scores in these areas to see if these are also major areas of concern for you. To the degree that they are also problems for you, addressing and treating depression should be a critical component of your pain self-management program.

Boredom is yet another aspect of depression and the chronic pain experience. The marriage between chronic pain and boredom is an awful one, and the offspring of this marriage is frequently depression. You may not be able to get rid of your pain, but you can certainly work on getting rid of the boredom. Working toward meaningful goals can help you find meaning in life again.

Thoughts of Ending It All: Suicide

People suffering from chronically painful conditions show elevated rates of suicidal thoughts and suicide attempts (Smith et al. 2004). I want you to go back to the Depression Scale and look at one particular item: "thoughts of harming yourself or 'ending it all.'" Many people who suffer from chronic pain have thoughts about not wanting to be around or wishing they wouldn't wake up in the morning. I hear this quite frequently from the people with whom I work. However, these thoughts can lead to planning or even attempting to end your life, so they must be taken seriously. It is important that you discuss your thoughts with a mental health care provider.

There is a critical distinction between passive thoughts about death and active suicidal thoughts, those that involve a sincere desire or intent to take your life. Ask yourself how close you have come to actually ending your life. Do you have plans, and do you know how you would do it? The closer you have come to ending your life, the more important it is that you seek help. See Resources for information about finding someone who can help, or call 9-1-1.

Treatment of Depression Related to Chronic Pain

Depression makes you feel like there is no hope. But depression lies. There are treatments available and experts you can turn to. Pain is bad enough; don't let yourself become depressed as well. Here are some ways you can change your experience now.

Physical Activity

Increasing your physical activity can reduce depression by releasing endorphins into your system, causing an overall sense of well-being. Exercise increases levels of neurotransmitters, including serotonin and GABA, which reduce pain and can ease depression. Exercise also helps to tire you out (in a good way), helping you get a better night's sleep and recharge your battery for the next day's activities. The bottom line: get moving.

Relaxation

By practicing various methods of relaxation, you can begin to cope more effectively with stressful situations and episodes of emotional suffering. Relaxation promotes increased energy, which in turn can reduce depression. Mind-body therapies and soothing treatments (such as massage and hot baths) can help shift your focus away from depressive thoughts and remind you that your body can be a source of pleasure, not just disappointment and pain.

A recent review of studies examining the utility of relaxation and hypnosis in pain management found that hypnosis and subsequent relaxation training produces significant decreases in pain (Jensen and Patterson 2006). These techniques can enhance your ability to cope with pain.

Cognitive Behavioral Therapy

Cognitive behavioral therapy focuses on problem solving, identifying unproductive thoughts and ideas about depression and pain, and developing adaptive coping strategies. Increasing pleasant activities and making behavioral changes can improve your mood. Cognitive behavioral therapy has been shown to be a solid, evidence-based treatment for mood problems and chronic pain. It can help you cope with depression, anxiety, and pain.

Antidepressant Medications

Antidepressants are frequently prescribed to assist with both mood problems (including depression) and pain conditions (including neuralgia, arthritis, low back pain, fibromyalgia, and central pain).

Despite their accepted and widespread use, we know surprisingly little about how antidepressants produce pain relief. However, it is thought that they improve mood and pain by modulating neurotransmitters like serotonin and norepinephrine (Jasmin et al. 2003).

Surprisingly, it is often the side effects of these medications that provide the most powerful improvements in the pain experience. For example, many antidepressants ease neuropathic pain sensations, and this is why they are frequently used by people suffering from headaches and nerve-generated pain conditions. Additionally, one of the side effects of some antidepressant medications is sedation, which can assist people suffering from sleep problems.

Goal Setting

Setting realistic, meaningful, and achievable goals can attack the core sense of failure and low self-esteem typified by depressive thoughts. Think back to exercise 4.7, Establish Your Goals, and exercise 10.11, Choose a Realistic Goal and Pace Yourself. Feel free to redraft your goals over and over as you read through this book and learn more about your unique pain issues.

Communication Training and Assertiveness Skills

Frequently, people with chronic pain tell me that as their pain drags on, everyone around them becomes a little less attentive and grows tired of their pain. Physicians and family members may even begin to pull away and appear to be frustrated.

A key pain management strategy is to develop your ability to express your wants and needs assertively. Improving communication skills, learning how to ask for what you want, and learning to be assertive can directly enhance your mood. You are simply more likely to get what you want and need if you can communicate to others what exactly that is.

What is assertive communication?   Assertive communication is simply asking for what you want or saying no to something you don't want in a very simple, direct, and honest fashion. The funny thing is that most people are assertive in some situations but not in others. For example, some people have no trouble standing up for others' rights but shy away from standing up for themselves. Some people will say no to someone who cuts in front of them in line at the store but will say nothing to their doctor if they feel misunderstood. Assertive communication is not being passive or submissive, which discounts your needs and puts others' needs first. Passive people may be seen as avoiders. But assertiveness is not about being aggressive, which involves demanding what you want in a hostile, angry, and accusatory manner. People who communicate aggressively end up being avoided by others. Communicating assertively is the middle ground, and it works. It can improve the quality of your relationships and help you feel better about yourself.

When to use assertive communication.   Use assertive communication when you want to share your feelings about something, make a request, or say no. Remember that other people are not mind readers; they do not know what is important to you or what is concerning you at any given moment. Think of being assertive as helping others know what you are feeling and what you need. You have the right to express yourself and ask for what you need. In his excellent book on assertive communication, *Your Perfect Right* (2001), Robert Alberti points out that standing up for yourself without guilt or apology and without disrespecting others is the key to assertive behavior.

How to communicate assertively. Assertive communication involves both verbal and nonverbal behaviors. Nonverbal assertive behaviors include maintaining good eye contact, remaining calm, and using positive body language (for instance, not moving away from the person you are talking to). Here is assertive communication in a nutshell:

1. Select a specific problem situation. For example, your physical therapist is late by twenty minutes each visit, and you don't get the help you need to learn the exercises.

2. Develop what you want to say ahead of time, using an I-statement. An I-statement could sound something like this: "I get frustrated that I cannot start my exercise program when you are late for my appointment." Practice this statement using good body language and a positive tone.

3. Follow up with a direct request. "How can we resolve this problem so that I can get all of the time I am scheduled for to practice my exercises?"

Pace yourself in practicing assertiveness skills, starting out gradually with less challenging situations. With small successes, your self-confidence will be enhanced. Then move on to more challenging situations.

Social Involvement

Pain is very isolating. You are never as alone as when you are in physical and emotional pain. Too many people with chronic pain spend most of their time in solitary pursuits: watching TV, playing video games, and so on. The mental distractions may be helpful for pain relief, but they don't provide the mental health benefits that social interactions can provide. Join a support group for people with pain; become a volunteer with an organization that's important to you. Do something that takes you back out into the world.

Enjoyable Activities

Pain often makes people stop doing things they once enjoyed. When they stop doing what they like to do, they suffer emotionally. But many people with chronic pain think they simply can't do what they used to do. They may stop doing just about everything. In reality, they may just need to modify the way they do things. As you learned in chapter 10, pacing, setting realistic goals, and modifying activities can help you to reconnect with pleasurable activities.

■ *Richard*

Richard was twenty-seven-years old when he injured his back falling from his delivery truck on a snowy day. He ended up with a three-level fusion of his lumbar region. It didn't take long for depression to set in. On the Depression Scale, he scored 4.5.

Richard's love had been bowling. He was quite good. And bowling played a major role in his social life. He had many buddies who also played on his league. But his surgeon told him he should never twist his torso—a motion essential to his seven-step hook. Richard believed he would never bowl again, and this belief only added to his depression.

As I worked with Richard, we broke down the behavioral tasks of bowling into small steps. To replace the seven-step hook, we got an okay from his physician and physical therapist to have him stand at the line and, using only arm motion, roll a straight ball. With this permission in mind, I convinced Richard to go back to his old stomping grounds: the bowling alley. But for now, he was not to even pick up a ball. He needed to take it slowly.

On Richard's first visit back to the bowling alley, he reconnected with friends who had not seen him since before his injury and surgeries. Just going back to the bowling alley lifted Richard's mood and reduced his depression.

Once Richard was used to being back at the bowling alley, I worked with him at modifying the tasks of bowling. We reduced the weight of his bowling ball, and he started playing only half a game, so that he was ending his game before his pain increased.

Several years later, Richard called to tell me that he had bowled an almost perfect game. He was still a good bowler. And since he no longer could drive a truck and make heavy deliveries, he changed his career: he bought the bowling alley's pro shop. He is now surrounded by friends, making a living, and his mood has greatly improved. Richard is no longer depressed; not surprisingly, he scored 0.8 on the Depression Scale the last time we met.

■ Steve

Steve had fibromyalgia that caused any movement of his muscles to be quite painful. He had a hard time even walking to the mailbox. He had once loved to fish—it was his ultimate joy—but he hadn't gone fishing in a very long time. He was afraid to walk down to the river, with the loose rocks and debris, and he had given up all hope of ever fishing again.

By the time Steve came to my practice, he was depressed and angry. (Keep in mind that both Steve and I live in Reno, Nevada, where the beautiful Truckee River runs right through the middle of town.) I asked Steve if he liked being around the river. Of course he did. Then I asked him if he would be willing to get up a little earlier the next morning (he had trouble sleeping anyway, like most people in pain) and get a cup of coffee, then park his car along the river facing east and watch the sun come up over the river. He wouldn't even have to leave his car.

At first he was hesitant, thinking being by the river would only remind him of what he was missing. But he tried it and was surprised by how much he enjoyed just listening to the water and watching the wind rustle the leaves in the trees. He reconnected with a love of the outdoors he had previously associated only with fishing. Even though his pain hadn't changed physically, he said he suffered a lot less that day.

ANXIETY

Like depression, anxiety often accompanies chronic pain. Anxiety and frustration have been shown to arise as a response to pain intensification, prolonged elevations in pain levels, or anticipation of increased pain (Fishban et al. 1997). Over time, the feelings of anxiety become such a part of the pain experience that you may have difficulty differentiating between pain and feelings of anxiety. Anxiety and emotional arousal caused by pain can also be heightened by stressful life events or daily hassles. While emotions do not cause pain, they do amplify it by either increasing pain intensity levels or undermining coping abilities.

Let's begin by taking a look at the extent to which you fear pain.

EXERCISE 11.3: FEAR OF PAIN SCALE

When your pain increases sharply, how concerned are you that

your pain will not settle down

not at all							very often
0	1	2	3	4	5	6	7

your pain will get even worse

not at all							very often
0	1	2	3	4	5	6	7

your pain will take a long time to calm down

not at all							very often
0	1	2	3	4	5	6	7

To score this exercise, add up the numbers you circled, then divide by 3. This is your fear of pain score. This number should be between 0 and 7. Put your score on the Pain Scorecard.

Interpreting Your Score

Your fear of pain score is a reflection of your anticipation of bad things to come with any increases in your pain.

Level three: 5.5 or more.   You are likely worried that your pain will take over and be with you for a long time. It's as if you are just waiting for the pain to start, and off and running your mind goes. A score at level three indicates that fear of pain is a major area of concern in your pain self-management program. Remember that many people with chronic pain are worried and fearful about their pain.

Level two: 3.4 to 5.4.   Your level of anticipatory fear about pain is similar to most people with chronic pain. You are moderately distressed by your fear of pain.

Level one: 3.3 or less.   You are not especially troubled by anticipatory worry and fear of pain. Pat yourself on the back, because anxiety and anticipation of pain does not seem to be a problem area in your pain management program.

EXERCISE 11.4: ANXIETY SCALE

Over the past two weeks, how often have you experienced the following symptoms?

shortness of breath

| not at all | | | | | | very often | |
| 0 | 1 | 2 | 3 | 4 | 5 | 6 | 7 |

racing heart

| not at all | | | | | | very often | |
| 0 | 1 | 2 | 3 | 4 | 5 | 6 | 7 |

frequent urination

| not at all | | | | | | very often | |
| 0 | 1 | 2 | 3 | 4 | 5 | 6 | 7 |

feeling tense and keyed up

| not at all | | | | | | very often | |
| 0 | 1 | 2 | 3 | 4 | 5 | 6 | 7 |

stomach distress

| not at all | | | | | | very often | |
| 0 | 1 | 2 | 3 | 4 | 5 | 6 | 7 |

trouble swallowing

| not at all | | | | | | very often | |
| 0 | 1 | 2 | 3 | 4 | 5 | 6 | 7 |

dizziness

| not at all | | | | | | very often | |
| 0 | 1 | 2 | 3 | 4 | 5 | 6 | 7 |

feeling shaky

| not at all | | | | | | very often | |
| 0 | 1 | 2 | 3 | 4 | 5 | 6 | 7 |

dry mouth

| not at all | | | | | | very often | |
| 0 | 1 | 2 | 3 | 4 | 5 | 6 | 7 |

cold hands

not at all   very often
0   1   2   3   4   5   6   7

trouble falling asleep

not at all   very often
0   1   2   3   4   5   6   7

trouble staying asleep

not at all   very often
0   1   2   3   4   5   6   7

racing thoughts

not at all   very often
0   1   2   3   4   5   6   7

To score this exercise, add up the numbers you circled, then divide by 13. This is your anxiety score. This number should be between 0 and 7. Place your score on the Pain Scorecard.

Interpreting Your Score

Level three: 3.1 or more.   Anxiety is a major component of your pain problem, and it is a major area of concern in your pain self-management program.

Level two: 1.6 to 3.0.   Your anxiety level is typical for a person with chronic pain. Your pain self-management program should include techniques for coping with anxiety.

Level one: 1.5 or less.   You have minimal problems with anxiety. This is not a major area of concern in your pain self-management program.

Chronic Pain and Anxiety

When people experience chronic pain, they typically get frustrated, anxious, upset, and overwhelmed, and they experience significant distress. Not knowing when the pain is going to get worse or how long a flare-up will last leads to a sense of vulnerability, futility, and uncertainty.

Difficulties falling asleep are often associated with anxiety (Morin 1993). Currie et al. (2000) found that people who describe themselves as poor sleepers reported higher levels of anxiety and depression.

Anxiety is the lighter fluid on the barbecue of life. You've got the hot coals (physical pain generators) just waiting to ignite. Add anxiety, and you have a major pain flare-up.

Anxiety includes fear of reinjury, anticipation of bad things to come, and plain old fear of pain. You may fear that the pain is going to keep escalating, getting worse and worse and ultimately becoming intolerable.

Coping with Anxiety During Flare-Ups

Here are some tips on coping with intense pain flare-ups coupled with high levels of anxiety:

- Alter your physical experience by taking a hot shower, applying a heating pad, rubbing the area, using ice, alternating heat and cold, applying pressure, using massage, or using TENS. Focus on the other sensations you experience rather than on pain.

- As early as possible in the pain flare-up, try to identify any triggers that may have set off this episode. The ideas and beliefs in the Fear of Pain Scale (*My pain will not settle down*, *My pain will get even worse*, and *My pain will take a long time to calm down*) are possible triggers. Challenge these ideas and test other possibilities such as *My pain has settled down in the past* and *It hasn't stayed bad forever* and *I can get through this.*

- Begin slow, deep breathing exercises and remind yourself to stay calm.

- Distract yourself: listen to music, do a crossword puzzle, watch TV, or play a video game.

- Use imagery. Imagine a block of ice resting on your pain site, visualize your endorphins activating and closing the door to pain, transfer your pain into a different sensation, such as numbness or dullness, and alter the quality of the experience.

Using Relaxation to Cope with Anxiety

No matter what your score on the Anxiety and Fear of Pain scales, relaxation can help you. Relaxation is the cornerstone of coping with anxiety. You cannot be relaxed and tense at the same time. You can't be calm and anxious at the same time. To escape the grip of anxiety, you need to learn ways to relax.

Most people (especially women) are chest breathers, meaning that they take shallow breaths using the muscles of the chest rather than the diaphragm. The reason this is important is related to the two nervous systems in the human body. The *sympathetic* system controls the fight-or-flight response. It activates the body in reaction to stress as a survival mechanism. It causes the heart rate to speed up and the muscles to tighten, ready to respond. When you become anxious, your sympathetic nervous system becomes active. The *parasympathetic* system helps calm the body down after a stressful situation. Chest breathing triggers the sympathetic nervous system. In order to calm anxiety, you need to activate the parasympathetic nervous system. The best way to do this is through diaphragmatic breathing, or belly breathing, which you learned in chapter 6.

ANGER

Anger can influence how you perceive pain (Suinn 2001). It can lower your tolerance to pain and be a major factor in pain flare-ups. Kerns, Rosenberg, and Jacob (1994) found that anger was highly correlated with pain perception and activity interference in a sample of male veterans.

There are several possible reasons for this connection between anger and pain. It may be that anger leads you to focus vigilantly on your body sensations and activates the sympathetic nervous system. Smith and Christensen (1992) suggest that anger leads to poor health habits such as use of alcohol, unhealthy diet, use of tobacco, disturbed sleep patterns, and poor compliance with doctors' recommendations—any of which can contribute to pain. There is strong evidence that anger is hazardous to your health and well-being.

Anger is a state of high emotional arousal, and you can deactivate the arousal of anger through relaxation skills. Think about a situation when your pain flared up, and then try to physically relax by using deep belly breathing, letting go, and releasing your body tension. Monitor your anger by retaking the Entitlement/Frustration Scale (exercise 8.6) weekly while you continue to practice relaxation techniques.

USING HUMOR TO RELIEVE DEPRESSION, ANXIETY, AND ANGER

I understand pain and suffering is serious stuff and not a laughing matter. However, humor can be useful to people in chronic pain, and I'd like to end this chapter about mood problems on a happy note.

Laughter is good medicine. No doubt about it. Laughing can cause your body to produce endorphins, and it increases the level of catecholamines in the blood, which can reduce inflammation (a frequent cause of pain). Unfortunately, the benefits of laughter are often unrecognized in those people who most need it: people with chronic pain.

When you use humor, you shift your perspective, which allows you to distance yourself from the immediate threat of a problem such as pain and view it from a slightly different frame of reference. This has the power to reduce the negative feelings that would typically occur. You may be better able to cope with your pain and find temporary relief by using laughter and humor. Research has shown a positive relationship between humor and increased pain tolerance (Nevo, Keinan, and Teshimovsky-Arditi 1993).

Berk (2001) cites the psychological benefits of humor based on quantitative and qualitative research. He found that humor reduces anxiety, tension, stress, depression, and loneliness; improves self-esteem; restores hope and energy; and provides a sense of empowerment and control. Humor can also reveal faulty thinking and expose ineffective ideas about pain.

I feel better after a good laugh with Jay Leno on *The Tonight Show*. Norman Cousins described in *Anatomy of an Illness as Perceived by the Patient* (W. W. Norton, 1979) how he used laughter and humor to deal with a crippling disease, degenerative ankylosing spondylitis. I recommend this book all the time to people in pain.

TO SUM UP

By now you realize the profound impact mood can have on your pain experience. Depression, anxiety, and humor are all part of your relationship with pain, and as such can be used to improve that relationship. With the help of the exercises, you should see what aspects of mood are influencing your pain and have some ideas as to how to improve your experience.

Mood has a huge impact on how you interact with others, as you will see more clearly in chapter 12, where we examine how your family affects your pain and how your pain affects your family.

All in the Family: The Social Implications of Chronic Pain

Chronic pain can hit couples, families, and significant others hard. When a family member suffers from chronic pain, the rest of the family is also caught up in the web of pain. This chapter will examine the effect your pain has had on the people close to you. This is an important aspect of the social component of the biopsychosocial phenomenon that is pain.

Frequently, when a person develops chronic pain, duties within the family are shifted. Chores may change. Others may have to pick up the slack. Resentments can build. To effectively manage the pain of the individual and the stress on the family, the focus must broaden to include everyone whose life is changed by the pain experience. The entire family needs to learn to live with the pain, not just the person designated the "patient."

Even though we are discussing your relationships with others, we still need to start with you. Let's look at your perceptions of how your pain affects other people.

EXERCISE 12.1: RELATIONSHIP INTERFERENCE SCALE

When your pain increases sharply, how concerned are you about the following?

your pain will negatively affect others

	not at all concerned					very concerned	
0	1	2	3	4	5	6	7

your pain will cause others to be upset

	not at all concerned					very concerned	
0	1	2	3	4	5	6	7

your pain will make others suffer

　　　　　not at all concerned　　　　　　　　　　　　　　　very concerned
　　　　0　　　1　　　2　　　3　　　4　　　5　　　6　　　7

your pain will interfere with the plans or activities of others

　　　　　not at all concerned　　　　　　　　　　　　　　　very concerned
　　　　0　　　1　　　2　　　3　　　4　　　5　　　6　　　7

your pain will bring everyone else down

　　　　　not at all concerned　　　　　　　　　　　　　　　very concerned
　　　　0　　　1　　　2　　　3　　　4　　　5　　　6　　　7

To score this exercise, add up all the numbers you circled, then divide by 5. This is your relationship interference score. This number should be between 0 and 7. Enter your score on the Pain Scorecard.

Interpreting Your Score

Your social interference score reflects your concerns about how your pain has affected others in your life, such as your family, friends, coworkers, and employer. This scale correlates with depression (exercise 11.2), catastrophizing about pain (exercise 8.1), and spousal criticism of pain (which you'll evaluate later in this chapter). I encourage you to look at your scores on these scales and see if this is true for you.

Level three: 4.2 or more.   You are quite worried about how your pain has affected others. This is a major component to your pain problem, and your pain self-management program should address this.

Level two: 2.1 to 4.1.   Your level of concern is typical for a person with chronic pain. This is an area of moderate concern for your pain self-management program.

Level one: 2.0 or less.   A level one score suggests minimal concern about how your pain has affected others. This is not an area of special concern in your self-management of pain.

PAIN, THE FAMILY, AND THE PAST

Pain truly is all in the family. Because the past informs the present, it is helpful to look back on how pain was dealt with in your family when you were growing up. When someone was hurt or had pain, what did your family do? How did they react? When you were ill or injured, did they become scared and take you to the emergency room? Did they simply tell you to grin and bear it? Or was their reaction somewhere in between? Did you ever care for someone who was hurt? How did your mother or father deal with sickness or painful accidents? This next exercise will help you answer these questions.

EXERCISE 12.2: REFLECT ON PAIN IN YOUR PAST

Take a few minutes to write out your thoughts and memories about pain in your family. Pay particular attention to what other people did. As you look back, did your family ignore pain, react within reason, or overreact to accidents and injuries?

HOW CHRONIC PAIN CAN AFFECT THE FAMILY

The effects on the families of those who suffer with chronic pain can be varied and intense. Let's take a closer look at some of the ways chronic pain can change family dynamics.

The person in pain often becomes the focus of attention, which may seem logical at first, but this can become a problem. When a family member suffers from chronic pain, the rest of the family feels it too. Management of your pain experience must include addressing the thoughts, feelings, and needs of the people close to you.

My experience tells me that most families can deal with someone in the family having short-term pain. An acute pain problem often does not disturb a family system. It is when pain becomes chronic and lasts longer than expected that the family unit becomes distressed.

Your family needs to have the opportunity to understand the nature and treatment of the pain. Uncertainty is stressful. Family members often search for a meaning of the pain, using their own experience as a lens through which to view your experience. Of course, no one can truly understand another's pain. Even people suffering from the same disease may experience it in vastly different ways.

Even when your feelings are apparent to you, they may not be clear to those around you. For example, depression and social withdrawal may be side effects of chronic pain. However, family members may interpret these changes as rejection. If you believe this is happening in your family, assistance from a family counselor or other mental health professional will be invaluable. Your family is worth it.

The stress of uncertainty is tough, but having no end to the pain in sight may be even tougher. The family needs to develop coping skills just as does the person in pain. You can reduce the level of distress for your entire family by addressing their concerns and teaching them how they can help you gain greater control over your pain experience. When their distress is reduced, people are more likely to make thoughtful, educated decisions.

If you suffer with chronic pain, you may find that family members become protective of you. They may take over your duties, discourage you from certain activities, and simply keep watch for anything they think might be harmful. Most of the time, when these family members take over your duties, they do not hand off any of their own responsibilities. The family member (usually a spouse or significant other) runs the risk of becoming overburdened.

As pain persists, you may see that loved ones have taken over household chores or financial responsibilities, or they may have cut back their activities to stay home with you. Roles can be reversed; others who have not had to work outside the home may now be forced to do so.

If you feel guilty about the demands you are already making on your family, you may begin to have difficulty being assertive about additional needs. You may even realize that you are using pain and pain behaviors as a way to get your needs met, rather than speaking up about these other needs. You can break this pattern by using a healthier, more effective alternative: assertive communication, which you learned about in the previous chapter.

EXERCISE 12.3: EVALUATE HOW YOUR PAIN AFFECTS YOUR FAMILY

It's easier to recognize how your family and loved ones are affected by your pain experience if you ask yourself a few questions about your activities and theirs. When you think "activities," think also "duties" or "chores." These may be in any of the following areas of life:

- Physical

- Emotional

- Vocational (work related)

- Sexual

- Recreational

- Social

- Spiritual

Now answer the following questions.

Have any of your typical activities, chores, or duties been altered or discontinued? If so, which ones?

Have others had to take on new chores, duties, or activities because of your pain problem? If so, which ones?

To what extent do other people encourage you to limit your activities, chores, or duties?

To what extent do other people encourage you to participate in activities, chores, or duties?

What does pain stop you from doing that you would otherwise like to be doing?

Who in your life (besides you) has had to change the most due to your pain?

PAIN MANAGEMENT HELPS THE WHOLE FAMILY

Effectively managing your pain can greatly improve the important relationships in your life. When you learn ways to better cope with your pain and show confidence in those skills, your family will feel less burdened and more optimistic. In other words, the better you learn to cope with your pain, the less burden there is on the people close to you. And because relationships are reciprocal, there is less burden on you.

USING PACING AS A SOCIAL TOOL

There are a variety of ways you can help your family (and yourself) in coping with the stresses and strains of chronic pain. Let's look at one of the most effective tools: pacing. Learning to pace yourself so that you are in less pain when others are present (for example, when your spouse or partner gets home from work) will make interactions more positive and successful. Being aware of when your pain is at its lowest during the day will help you choose (to the extent that you can) the best time to spend time with family. Timing your medications for effective pain relief can also give you the opportunity for better interactions with others.

Planning ahead is the bedrock of pacing. For example, when you go somewhere with your sister, let her know that it's possible you may want to leave earlier than she will, and suggest that you take separate cars. Or, if you go to the movie theater, consider getting there early to get a seat in the back or on an aisle, so you can get up and move around if necessary without bothering others. This will give you a personal sense of control, and it may make the social event more pleasant and enjoyable for you and for others.

Pacing yourself is tough enough when it comes to doing chores, but when you are having fun, it is even harder. It is also even more important. The danger is that you will get caught up in the moment, overdo it, and then pay a big price.

If you can find the willpower to leave an enjoyable situation while you are still feeling good, you can begin to change one important lesson pain may have taught you: the pairing of "the more I do" and "the more I hurt." As you know by now, breaking this link is very important to your recovery. When you stop before your pain flares up, you learn to associate activity with reduced pain.

HOW YOUR FAMILY THINKS ABOUT AND REACTS TO YOUR PAIN

What you think about reinjury, control, harm, depression, anger, doctors, medications, and the like affects how you feel. Your family's thoughts about these issues matter, too. Do any of the following sound familiar?

Just rest. You don't want to make your pain worse.

Stop that! You could hurt yourself.

We can't expect you to do anything since you are in pain.

You are making more of this pain than you need to.

You shouldn't be in as much pain as you say you are.

You should rest and lie down when you are in pain.

Stop and let me do that.

While all the above statements are common, that does not make them right. Nor does it make them at all helpful—to you or to others. Not surprisingly, the stress and work of helping to care for someone suffering from chronic pain can lead to poor health for the helper. So we need to make some positive changes for both you and your loved ones.

Pain as a Way of Communicating Your Needs

Pain may become a means for expressing needs unrelated to the pain experience. Because pain can disrupt important relationships, you may attempt to use the pain experience to obtain what the pain has taken away: the attention and caring of others. While this may be normal, it can become problematic for the relationship if pain becomes your primary way of getting your needs met.

Pain Behaviors Versus Wellness Behaviors

In chapter 9, I addressed the concept of pain behaviors, those actions that communicate to others that you are hurting. (Remember that pain behaviors include both verbal and nonverbal communication:

grimacing, bracing yourself when you walk, crying, and telling others you hurt.) Whatever your pain behaviors, you wouldn't do them if they were not reinforced in some way. In other words, your pain behaviors are the most effective things you have learned to do when you are experiencing pain. However, sometimes these behaviors become problems in themselves.

One of the most common sources of reinforcement of your pain behaviors is the people closest to you. For better or worse, the actions of others—intentional or not—are quite likely influencing your pain experience. It is human nature to continue behavior that is rewarded and discontinue behavior that is somehow punished. If your family becomes sympathetic and helpful every time you limp, you are much more likely to limp. If your family becomes sympathetic and helpful every time you do your physical therapy without limping, you are much more likely to do your physical therapy without limping.

Reactions to Pain

An important influence on your coping and adjustment to pain is the reaction of your partner and family. Sometimes, family members react to a person's pain with irritation or disbelief. Other times, people react by becoming overly solicitous. The best possible reaction is one that encourages you to think and act in ways that contribute to your well-being. Let's take a closer look at each of these possibilities.

Invalidation

It is quite disturbing to be in pain and have others not believe you or think you are making more of it than necessary. When you are in pain, your family may get annoyed and irritated with you. Because your pain is mostly invisible, others may think it isn't such a big deal. Caring partners and others can grow tired of a family pain problem if it lasts for more than a few weeks. When you feel invalidated in your pain experience, your suffering increases, especially when the person by whom you feel invalidated is a family member.

Let's take a look at the extent to which you feel criticized about your pain. For the remainder of this section, I will use the term "partner" to refer to your spouse, significant other, or other important family member. You know who you are referring to with this one term.

EXERCISE 12.4: PARTNER CRITICISM OF PAIN SCALE

Rate how frequently your partner does the following things. Then check the box whether you dislike it or like it when he or she does those things.

complains that your pain has made his/her life difficult

not at all   very often
0   1   2   3   4   5   6   7   dislike ☐   like ☐

gets irritated or angry at you because of your pain

not at all   very often
0   1   2   3   4   5   6   7   dislike ☐   like ☐

gets upset with you for taking too much pain medication

not at all   very often

0   1   2   3   4   5   6   7   dislike ☐   like ☐

becomes irritated with you for not getting better

not at all   very often

0   1   2   3   4   5   6   7   dislike ☐   like ☐

criticizes you for not increasing your physical activity

not at all   very often

0   1   2   3   4   5   6   7   dislike ☐   like ☐

gets mad at you when you tell him/her you are in pain

not at all   very often

0   1   2   3   4   5   6   7   dislike ☐   like ☐

nags you about being more active when you recline, sit, or lie around the house

not at all   very often

0   1   2   3   4   5   6   7   dislike ☐   like ☐

tells you that you should not be in as much pain as you say you are

not at all   very often

0   1   2   3   4   5   6   7   dislike ☐   like ☐

To score this exercise, add up the numbers you circled, then divide by 8. This is your partner criticism of pain score. This number should be between 0 and 7. Place your score in the Pain Scorecard.

Interpreting Your Score

As you might guess, the experiences listed above are not very common among people who suffer from chronic pain, and this is good.

Level three: 1.8 or more.   Your partner is seriously struggling with your pain problem. You are in trouble, and so is your partner. It's unpleasant to feel that someone is criticizing or discouraging some aspect of your pain, so most likely you checked "dislike" for these items. If you scored at level three, your partner should be included in your pain treatment plan. Relationship distress is contributing to your pain experience.

Level two: 0.5 to 1.7.   You definitely have some problems with your partner, and this needs to be addressed.

Level one: 0.4 or less.   A score in this range suggests that your partner expresses minimal criticism, anger, and frustration with your pain problem, and this bodes well for your relationship. Your chronic pain problem has not damaged your relationship significantly.

Tips for addressing critical responses.   If an important relationship is distressed because of your pain problem, try these steps to improve it:

- Discuss with your family what your actual medical diagnosis is. They need to know your pain generators—the physical reasons for your pain. If the doctors have not found a specific reason for your pain, this will be hard not only on you but also on your family. Seek the best medical opinion about your condition and discuss it with your family. (For more on this topic, see chapter 5.)

- Discuss with your family what ideas they have about the nature of your pain diagnosis. What are they worried could be the reason for your pain? Is the cause of your pain catastrophic, like cancer or a tumor? Or does your family have no clue why you are experiencing pain? Do they believe you are overreacting to your pain? You need to ask these questions and know the answers.

- Sometimes, family members may feel as if pain is being used to manipulate them. You need to be aware of this possibility and ask the people in your life if they feel this way. Ask yourself, *Is there any possible benefit I am getting from my pain?* or *Can I imagine that someone else would think I am getting something from my pain, and if so, what would that be?*

- Some assertiveness training may be beneficial for you in order to help you state your needs more directly.

Solicitousness

Another possible reaction your partner may have to your pain is solicitousness, or extreme care and concern tinged with protectiveness and apprehensiveness. It's nice to have a partner who cares about you and is there for you when your pain flares up. Your partner's concern may make you feel loved. However, as you'll see, solicitousness has some potential pitfalls.

Let's evaluate whether solicitousness is a dynamic in your relationship.

EXERCISE 12.5: PARTNER REINFORCEMENT OF PAIN SCALE

Rate how frequently your partner does the following. Then check the box whether you dislike it or like it when he or she does those things.

pays more attention to your needs when you are in pain than when you're not in pain

not at all   very often
0   1   2   3   4   5   6   7   dislike ☐   like ☐

encourages you to rest when you're in pain

not at all   very often

0   1   2   3   4   5   6   7   dislike ☐   like ☐

is especially nice to you when you are in pain

not at all   very often

0   1   2   3   4   5   6   7   dislike ☐   like ☐

gives you a massage when you're in pain

not at all   very often

0   1   2   3   4   5   6   7   dislike ☐   like ☐

brings you your pain medication when you're in pain

not at all   very often

0   1   2   3   4   5   6   7   dislike ☐   like ☐

asks you how you feel when you're in pain

not at all   very often

0   1   2   3   4   5   6   7   dislike ☐   like ☐

asks if he/she can help in some way when you're in pain

not at all   very often

0   1   2   3   4   5   6   7   dislike ☐   like ☐

encourages you to call your doctor when your pain flares up

not at all   very often

0   1   2   3   4   5   6   7   dislike ☐   like ☐

takes over your chores and duties when you are in pain

not at all   very often

0   1   2   3   4   5   6   7   dislike ☐   like ☐

To calculate your score for this exercise, add up the numbers you circled, then divide by 9. This is your partner's reinforcement of pain score. This number should be between 0 and 7. Enter your score on the Pain Scorecard.

Interpreting Your Score

Remember that this is *your* score and *your* appraisal of your partner. This is your perception. It may or may not reflect reality. You'll need to discuss these scores with your partner in order to confirm your conclusions.

Level three: 4.5 or more.   Reinforcement of pain is a significant area of concern. If you checked "like" for many of these items, your partner's solicitous behavior may be serving to reward your pain behaviors. While this may feel good, in the long run it may be problematic for your pain self-management program. But if you dislike extra attention when you are in pain, your partner's actions are probably not reinforcing your pain behaviors.

You may need to explore what your partner believes is the cause of your pain. This will influence the way he or she treats you. It's possible that your partner believes your diagnosis is catastrophic and therefore wants to take care of you.

High scores on this scale have been associated with high marital satisfaction. This is obviously a good thing, right? Maybe not. High levels of reinforcement of pain have been associated with high reported pain levels, high frequency of pain behaviors, and greater perceived disability on the part of the person in pain as well. This may lead to reduced activity levels, more help-seeking behaviors, and the use of fewer or less effective coping strategies (Romano et al. 1995).

Level two: 2.6 to 4.4.   If you scored within the average range on this scale, your partner is apparently acting in a caring way. However, spousal attention—if it becomes solicitous—may be too much of a good thing.

Level one: 2.5 or less.   A score at this level suggests that your partner is not reinforcing your pain behaviors. This is positive in terms of pain management goals, but it could also mean that you are getting no affirmation of your pain experience.

It is imperative that family members learn to reinforce only helpful behaviors (exercise, movement, and positive attitudes) and not inadvertently reinforce problem behaviors. It's best if the people around you simply ignore behaviors associated with the "sick" or "victim" role (lying in bed, resting for long periods of time, or taking a lot of medications).

Reinforcement can affect much more than just behavior, however. Many people in pain report more disability and more severe pain associated with times when their families or partners act solicitously. And it's not just a matter of perception.

In a 1995 study by Flor and colleagues, researchers delivered electric shocks to subjects in the presence of their spouses/significant others and had those subjects rate their pain. Among subjects who reported their spouses or significant others as being solicitous, the subjects rated (perceived) their pain as more severe in the presence of their spouses or significant others. But that's not all. EKGs also showed a larger response to the shock. Researchers did not see the same results in subjects who did not list their partners as solicitous. The "help" of these solicitous spouses had actually conditioned the subjects to feel pain more strongly.

Tips for modifying solicitous responses.   If you scored in level two or three on the Partner Reinforcement of Pain Scale, you may want to work with your partner to modify the solicitous behavior. Here are a few tips to get you started:

- Explain to your partner that the solicitous behaviors (as much as they are appreciated) may serve as inadvertent cues for increased pain behavior.

- Redirect expressions of concern to the reinforcement of wellness behaviors. Ask your partner to give you a massage after you take a short walk rather than when your pain is at its worst. This reinforces the activity of walking. Instead of getting your pain pills for you, your partner can get you a book so you can distract yourself from the pain.

- Suggest ways your partner can step back and let you do a little more (such as taking out a small bag of garbage or doing the dishes) when you are not in pain.

- Your partner can be encouraged and given permission to ignore pain behavior and instead focus on your progress and give positive feedback. Try saying "I really appreciate it when you ask how I am feeling when I am bracing myself or have trouble getting out of the chair, but I would rather you remind me of the progress I have made in my stretching and exercise program."

- Provide family members with information about the cause of your pain.

- Ask your partner to give other supportive responses that are not solicitous: for example, distracting you or suggesting that you relax.

You may also want to share these instructions with friends and relatives who habitually focus conversations on pain and suffering. You could say something along the lines of "Because I have had this pain for so long, I want to give you permission to talk to me about anything other than my pain and disability." My clinical experience tells me that your friends and family often don't know what else to talk about and feel grateful and relieved to have permission to relate to you on issues other than pain. The goal here is to increase your control, function, and independence.

Is Your Family Supporting You in Wellness?

Let's end this chapter with two exercises that will help you evaluate how effectively your partner is supporting you in wellness.

EXERCISE 12.6: PARTNER DISCOURAGEMENT OF WELLNESS SCALE

Rate how frequently your partner does the following. Then check whether you dislike it or like it when he or she does those things.

becomes irritated with you when you try to increase your physical activity

not at all   very often

0   1   2   3   4   5   6   7   dislike ☐   like ☐

cautions you about reinjuring yourself when you are physically active (for example, exercising, working around the yard, walking)

not at all   very often

0   1   2   3   4   5   6   7   dislike ☐   like ☐

warns you when you are physically active, "You'll pay the price if you keep that up"

not at all   very often

0   1   2   3   4   5   6   7   dislike ☐   like ☐

stops you from doing physical activities that could increase your pain

not at all   very often

0   1   2   3   4   5   6   7   dislike ☐   like ☐

To calculate your score for this exercise, add up the numbers you circled, then divide by 4. This is your partner discouragement of wellness score. This number should be between 0 and 7. Place your score on the Pain Scorecard.

Interpreting Your Score

Level three: 4.4 or more.   Your partner is expressing significant concern that could interfere with your recovery. He or she is not supporting your efforts to engage in movement, and over the long haul, this will be problematic for you.

Your partner is likely worried that you may engage in activities that will cause a major pain flare-up or reinjure you, leading to problems not only for you but for the entire family—including your partner. You may want to talk to your partner about this issue, perhaps asking, "How bad is it for you when I am in pain?" or "What is the worst part of my pain problem for you?" Your partner may experience high levels of distress and develop a "protector" role that ultimately works against your recovery.

If you dislike it when your partner tries to stop you from being physically active, you will need to discuss this. Keep in mind that if your partner is actually cautioning you about doing things that could cause harm and injury, such as lifting or carrying too much weight or working too long without appropriate rest, his or her concerns are warranted and should be heeded. However, if your partner tells you to stop or warns you that you will hurt yourself no matter what you are doing—even when you are pacing yourself well and engaging in activities that are not deemed harmful to you—you will need to share with your partner what you are learning in this book about proper activity pacing, good body mechanics, and so on.

Level two: 2.3 to 4.3.   A score in this range suggests that your partner is somewhat worried about you overdoing activities. The discussion and suggestions above may be helpful.

Level one: 2.2 or less.   Your partner is not discouraging your wellness activities. This is a good thing.

Tips to help family members support your pain management.   You can help your loved ones help you. Here are some ideas:

- Tell them about the rationale for your new way of thinking about and managing your pain. Explain chronic versus acute pain, the gate-control theory of pain, and the bio-psychosocial model.

- Share with them the coping skills you are learning in this book, including attention diversion skills (distraction), activity-based skills (activity pacing and deep breathing), and cognitive strategies (challenging catastrophic ideas, remembering that hurt does not equal harm).

- Work with your family to improve communication skills and set mutual goals. Consider having regular family meetings to review progress and get feedback about what is and is not working.

- Schedule visits with family, friends, and health care providers so that you are at your best. If your pain is worse in the evening, ask people to visit in the morning or early afternoon. If you feel groggy twenty minutes after taking your pain medication, plan activities, appointments, and visits for later.

EXERCISE 12.7: PARTNER REINFORCEMENT OF WELLNESS SCALE

Rate how frequently your partner does the following. Then check whether you dislike it or like it when he or she does those things.

encourages you to do your chores and duties

not at all   very often
0   1   2   3   4   5   6   7   dislike ☐   like ☐

tells you he/she likes it when you increase your physical activity

not at all   very often
0   1   2   3   4   5   6   7   dislike ☐   like ☐

pays attention to you when you are physically active (for example, doing chores around the house or yard)

not at all   very often
0   1   2   3   4   5   6   7   dislike ☐   like ☐

pushes you to be more active

not at all   very often
0   1   2   3   4   5   6   7   dislike ☐   like ☐

tells you that he/she appreciates it when you help around the house or yard

not at all   very often

0   1   2   3   4   5   6   7   dislike ☐   like ☐

encourages you to walk and exercise

not at all   very often

0   1   2   3   4   5   6   7   dislike ☐   like ☐

To calculate your score for this exercise, add up the numbers you circled, then divide by 6. This is your partner reinforcement of wellness score. This number should be between 0 and 7. Place your score on the Pain Scorecard. This is a reverse-scored scale, so in this case, higher scores are better.

Interpreting Your Score

Level three: 2.3 or less.   Your partner is not taking advantage of opportunities to reward you with positive attention for engaging in healthy activities. You may want to ask your partner to help support your efforts to become more active (for example, by going with you on walks or exercising together).

Level two: 2.4 to 4.0.   You are getting a level of encouragement that is within the average range for people with chronic pain.

Level one: 4.1 or more.   Your partner is doing a wonderful job paying positive attention to your wellness activities. This is especially true if you said you like it when he or she reinforces your efforts to be as active as you can. Give your partner a high five and say thanks for helping you get better.

If you dislike it when your partner encourages you in your wellness behaviors, ask yourself what it is about that particular behavior that you dislike. Perhaps you feel like your partner is pushing you too hard to be more active, but maybe you are too inactive. Remember the importance of activity pacing. Doing too little or too much is a problem. Also, remember that your partner's behavior can play a major role in your participation in activity when you're in pain and your willingness to continue to engage in these activities.

EXERCISE 12.8: START THE CONVERSATION

Have your partner read this chapter of the book. If you or your partner have difficulty discussing your relationship dynamics, try underlining a few important sentences in the book before you give it to your partner to read. You may even want to include notes in the margins. You could write on the side of the page, "What do you think about this?" as one way of inviting your partner's comments.

TO SUM UP

You should now have a better understanding of how you and the people around you interact about your pain and how this affects your experience of pain. Your past, how pain was treated in your family, may have affected how you deal with pain now as well as how you expect your pain to be interpreted and dealt with by others. But these may not be the healthiest assumptions or expectations you could have.

It is important to understand how your family feels about your pain by looking at how you are treated in the context of pain. The exercises in this chapter helped you better understand how your pain experience is affecting your family. That understanding can help you figure out how your family's experience of your pain affects you.

Many of the ideas you've explored in this chapter are relevant to other parts of your life outside the family—particularly your work. The same dynamics that arise between you and your family can happen with your employer and your coworkers. And you can use the same approaches—for instance, using assertive communication and seeking out the other person's point of view—to improve those relationships.

Chapter 13 is about sex—one of the most physical activities involved in a relationship. As important as sex is to a relationship, it is equally as important to your physical well-being.

CHAPTER 13

Sex

Pain affects the social lives of those suffering beneath its weight. You may already know that there is virtually no part of your life not changed by chronic pain. But one of the aspects of that social life is sex. And too often, this important subject goes unaddressed.

HOW CHRONIC PAIN CAN CHANGE SEX

No matter how strong your relationship, chronic pain can come between you and your partner. Look back to exercise 10.7, the Interference and Avoidance Scale for Personal Care Activities. Check your "before" and "now" scores for sexual activity. Has this score remained unchanged, or has sex decreased in frequency? Most often, pain decreases sexual activity. There are several possible reasons for this. Your partner may be afraid of hurting you. You may be afraid of being hurt. Your pain medications may decrease libido. Constantly fighting chronic pain can be exhausting. Tired people tend to experience a decrease in libido (ask any new parent). And let's not forget the shadowy hobgoblin of depression. Depression interferes with satisfaction and quality of sexual functioning, although it does not necessarily limit the drive and frequency of sexual activities.

Chronic pain may change the way you see the world, but it also changes the way the world sees you. This includes the people who know you best. Family members (including your spouse or lover) may no longer see you in the same way they did before your pain began. Your roles within the family may change, including your role in your sexual relationship. Whereas you may have initiated sex in the past, you may be hesitant to now, fearing that sex will make you hurt more (which may or may not be true). Or your partner may have once seen you as active and healthy and now see you as injured or a patient. He or she may be afraid of hurting you or afraid that activity will worsen your pain or trigger a flare-up. Fear of pain can lead partners to pull away from each other; no one wants to cause someone else pain. In addition, you may feel guilty for being unable to have a normal sexual relationship with your partner.

Whatever the reason, a decrease in sexual activities is not a good thing if you once enjoyed that part of your life. Past pleasures are replaced with frustration and conflict. This is the cruelest part of chronic pain. It is no surprise that many people with chronic pain resent the changes that pain brings.

TALKING ABOUT SEX

Talking about sex is still uncomfortable for many people—even some in the health care professions. You may not be comfortable talking about sex with your physician. Your physician may not be comfortable talking about sex with you. But someone needs to be talking about it. It's your pain. If chronic pain is damaging your sex life, talk to your physician or anyone else on your pain care team with whom you feel comfortable.

Odds are, you're not talking about sex with your partner either. Perhaps you don't want to do anything to hurt your partner, so you don't want to push it. But that can be perceived as lack of interest and can be a step back. When one partner feels rejected, it can be confusing and depressing.

The flip side is that there are instances where people use pain to communicate things they don't want to say. Saying you hurt is a way to keep your partner away. But this may be a communication issue, not a pain issue. People may use pain as a way to skirt issues like intimacy and trust. Pain behaviors often say "Stay away from me" and serve as a way to avoid real assertiveness.

TAKING BACK YOUR SEX LIFE

Many people with chronic pain have not had sexual contact with their partner for months or years due to the pain problem. They talk about the fears they have or their partner has that sex will cause more pain. They miss the intimacy and the caring and the touching. Part of the problem is that some people think that all caring behaviors lead to sexual intercourse. This all-or-nothing thinking leads to the conclusion that any touching or romance will lead to increased pain through sexual intercourse. This problematic way of thinking is yet another example of the tremendous influence your thoughts and ideas can have on your life.

You can decide that pain will not destroy your relationships, and you can take back your life—including your sex life. It comes down to restoring positive relations with your partner. I encourage you both to read this chapter. Simply by doing so, you are already moving toward improving your relationship and showing how important your partner is.

This exercise will help you take a realistic look at the impact your pain is having on your sex life.

EXERCISE 13.1: GET REAL WITH PAIN AND SEX

Does pain interfere with your sexual ability or your frequency of sexual activity?

With whom have you talked about sexual problems?

How did you feel about talking about sex?

Has your interest in sex changed? If so, how?

If your interest has changed, why do you think this is?

Has your partner's interest changed?

If your partner's interest has changed, why do you think this is? Ask him or her.

Have the changes in your sex life brought on by chronic pain stressed your relationship?

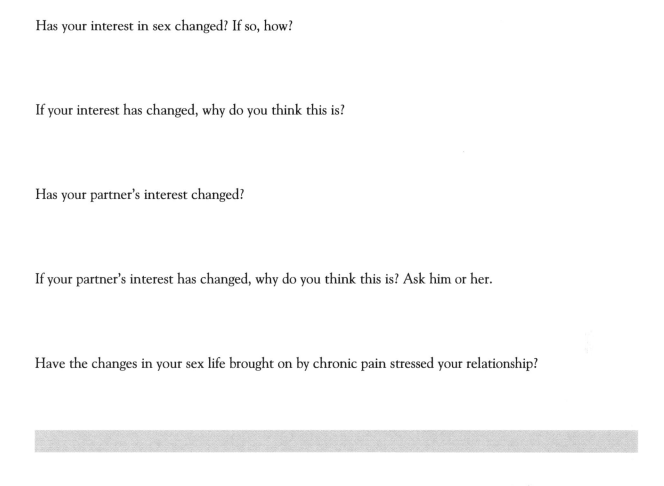

TREATMENT ISSUES

If you aren't satisfied with your sex life, there are a number of issues to think about. Here are two of the most important.

First, sex is a physical act that requires physical functioning. But pain does not limit your sensuality, your capacity for enjoying the pleasures of the senses. This is an important distinction. You can lose the enjoyment of the experience if you are too caught up with "performing" physically.

Second, keep in mind that you are not the only one having a problem with sex; so is your partner. Open communication is the key to restoring sexual relations. Start by agreeing that you will be committed to making your relationship a priority. Learn how pain can affect sexual activity. Then try implementing some of the suggestions that follow.

Treatment Suggestions

Here are some ways to repair your relationship and reclaim your sex life:

■   Find ways to focus on intimacy and sensuality when sex is out of the question. Think back to the kinds of things you did in the courtship phase of your relationship. Think *romance*.

- ▪ Approach sex when your pain is tolerable. Engage in sexual activity at times of the day when pain is at its lowest. Use your Discovery Journal (from chapter 4) to figure out that time for you.

- ▪ Sexual activity can be planned to coincide with the peak action of medications. If you don't know when that is, monitor the effectiveness of your medication throughout each day for a week.

- ▪ Move. Get used to moving. Conditioning through exercise can help you maintain your energy during sexual activity.

- ▪ Relax. Shared pleasure is heightened when both partners are relaxed and approach encounters with some thought to pacing, going slowly, and adopting an attitude of playfulness.

- ▪ Think about an atmosphere that will create a sensuous mood for both of you, and plan to make it happen.

- ▪ Experiment with more comfortable positions. Bring in props such as pillows to support the parts of the body that hurt when moved.

- ▪ Agree on a strategy about how each of you will deal with pain.

- ▪ Plan a date—a time when you can focus on your relationship.

TO SUM UP

Sex is not a luxury. It is an important part of life, especially for those in committed relationships. Don't let embarrassment or awkwardness keep you from discussing sex with those who can help you. This chapter has given you some insight and tools to help you improve your enjoyment of one of nature's greatest gifts.

Of course, one of the people with whom you should discuss sex and pain is your doctor. Ideally, your relationship with your doctor would be open and honest, but reality sometimes falls short. Chapter 14 examines the many and varied issues that can crop up in communicating with your doctor.

CHAPTER 14

Working with Your Doctors

Physicians who specialize in working with people with chronic pain want to help their patients feel less pain. This is important to mention because this chapter is focused on physician behavior as seen through your eyes, the eyes of the person experiencing pain, and it's possible that certain actions taken by your physicians may have inadvertently worked against your recovery process. This does not mean you should ignore the recommendations of physicians or avoid seeing them. It simply means that you need to look carefully at your relationships with your doctors and your feelings about the care you've received.

You experience pain not in a vacuum but within a social context. This means that you do not experience pain alone. It occurs around other people, including the physicians who treat you. This chapter focuses on your perception of what your physicians have done to help you in your pain management. Remember that a major goal of this book is to help you discover what is perpetuating, exacerbating, and maintaining your pain problem.

Most medical professionals get about ten hours of pain management training in their entire medical education. So while they are experts in medicine, they may not be experts in chronic pain, and they certainly are not experts in *your* chronic pain. You are.

A TEAM APPROACH TO PAIN MANAGEMENT

People with chronic pain who feel they have not been listened to or comprehensively evaluated are likely to respond with greater fears of pain, have more negative interactions with health care providers, and catastrophize about their pain. Until they feel that everything that should be done medically has been done, their pain management rehabilitation will be stymied.

Researchers have found that treatment satisfaction was negatively correlated with depression, reported number of physicians consulted, and number of physician visits twelve months after treatment (McCracken 1997). In other words, the more physicians you have consulted, and the more times you have visited them, the more depressed and less satisfied you are a year after treatment.

It is most helpful for you to see yourself as a partner with your physicians and any other health care professionals working with you (such as physical therapists, psychologists, occupational therapists, pharmacists, nurse case managers, and nutritionists). In fact, you will benefit most if you view these people as a team of specialists who are working to assist you in coping more effectively with your pain. Just remember that you are a member of that team.

The effectiveness of your medical treatment depends partly on the interpersonal context in which it takes place—that is, it depends upon the relationship you have with your physician and other members of your team. A wide body of research suggests that a stressful interaction with your physician has a negative impact on your health. My research and that of others has shown that the effectiveness of your pain management is influenced by your personal characteristics, the unique interaction you have with your physician, and your physician's background, training, and personality.

Here are three exercises to help you evaluate your experiences with your physicians and understand what effect these experiences have had on your pain. In these exercises, think about the overall experience you have had with all your doctors since you developed pain, rather than focusing on one or two positive or negative experiences. However, you can complete any of the exercises a second time with only one physician in mind to evaluate that individual relationship.

EXERCISE 14.1: PHYSICIAN REINFORCEMENT OF WELLNESS SCALE

My doctors have talked to me about different ways to manage my pain besides taking medication, resting, and receiving shots.

not at all   very often
0   1   2   3   4   5   6   7

My doctors have tried to get me to exercise and be more physically active.

not at all   very often
0   1   2   3   4   5   6   7

My doctors have tried to include me as a participant in my own health care such as giving me choices, asking for my feedback, and encouraging me to develop certain skills, such as muscle stretching, that I could practice on my own.

not at all   very often
0   1   2   3   4   5   6   7

When I have tried to increase my physical activity in the past, my doctors have encouraged me to continue.

not at all   very often
0   1   2   3   4   5   6   7

To score this exercise, add up the numbers you circled, then divide by 4. This is your physician reinforcement of wellness score. This number should be between 0 and 7. Place your score on your Pain Scorecard. This is a reverse-scored scale, so higher scores are better.

Interpreting Your Score

Level three: 2.0 or less. You have a right to ask your doctors why they fear normal activities are going to aggravate your pain and why they perhaps have not included you in the treatment planning. Your physician may have medical justification for discouraging you from certain activities. It's also possible that your doctors have not talked enough with you about what you should and shouldn't be doing. You would benefit from asking your physicians about each of the items on this scale to see if you could be taking a more active role in your rehabilitation.

Level two: 2.1 to 3.9. You are within the average range of experiences with physicians for most people who are in chronic pain.

Level one: 4.0 or more. Your physicians are doing a wonderful job reinforcing wellness activities. They have likely followed an evidence-based model in your pain management, and you are getting the benefit of this approach.

My research on this topic has suggested that people who score high on physician reinforcement of wellness also have lower levels of catastrophizing about their pain. This makes sense in that they are being included as a partner in their pain management and can exercise more control over their efforts to manage their pain.

EXERCISE 14.2: PHYSICIAN DISCOURAGEMENT OF WELLNESS SCALE

My doctors have warned me against doing anything that could make my pain worse, even after six months following the onset of my pain and/or any surgery for my pain.

not at all						very often	
0	1	2	3	4	5	6	7

Even after six months following the onset of my pain and/or any surgery for my pain, I have been cautioned by doctors that serious injury or paralysis could result if I attempt to increase my physical activity.

not at all						very often	
0	1	2	3	4	5	6	7

Even after six months following the onset of my pain and/or any surgery for my pain, my doctors have continued to recommend that I restrict most of my physical activities.

not at all						very often	
0	1	2	3	4	5	6	7

Even after six months following the onset of my pain and/or any surgery for my pain, my doctors have told me "you might harm yourself if you attempt to increase your physical activity."

not at all						very often	
0	1	2	3	4	5	6	7

My doctors have gotten annoyed at me for exploring alternative treatments for managing my pain (such as relaxation training, nutritional education, and stress management).

not at all   very often
0   1   2   3   4   5   6   7

To score this exercise, add up the numbers you circled, then divide by 5. This is your physician discouragement of wellness score. This number should be between 0 and 7. Place your score in your Pain Scorecard.

Interpreting Your Score

Level three: 2.9 or more.   Your physician is sending a strong message that you should stay inactive and take it slow. I strongly suggest you ask your physician about the recommendation that you restrict your activities. Being cautious about overdoing activities makes good medical sense, and by now, you understand the importance of activity pacing. However, discouraging appropriate levels of activity is counterproductive and goes against all recent research on the topic of movement and chronic pain.

My research suggests that when physicians discourage wellness in people with chronic pain, the people in pain often have greater fears of re injury. Sometimes, physicians can inadvertently reinforce your pain problem by being overly cautious and prescribing inactivity long after healing has taken place. This approach may indirectly foster dysfunction and disability. There may be a good reason for your doctor to recommend restricted activity, but you need to find out what that reason is.

Doctors can sometimes also foster dependency, by writing prescriptions for drugs, performing procedures, running medical tests, and providing surgeries. Excessive visits to a doctor can train you to hope for a solution, cure, or fix, even when none is possible. Be sure to discuss with your physician the reasons for all tests, procedures, and office visits. Ask questions about your prognosis and get the information you need to keep your expectations reasonable.

Level two: 1.4 to 2.8.   Your physician may be worried about you overdoing activities and placing yourself in harm's way. The suggestions for level three scores may be helpful to you.

Level one: 1.3 or less.   Your physicians are not discouraging you from taking an active role in your rehabilitation, and this is positive.

EXERCISE 14.3: PHYSICIAN CRITICISM OF PAIN SCALE

My doctors have said they cannot find anything physically wrong that would explain why I continue to have pain.

not at all   very often
0   1   2   3   4   5   6   7

I have had doctors tell me I should not be in as much pain as I say I am.

not at all							very often
0	1	2	3	4	5	6	7

My doctors have accused me of exaggerating my pain.

not at all							very often
0	1	2	3	4	5	6	7

My doctors have gotten annoyed at me when I've complained of pain.

not at all							very often
0	1	2	3	4	5	6	7

My doctors have criticized me for not increasing my physical activity.

not at all							very often
0	1	2	3	4	5	6	7

My doctors have told me that the pain is all in my head (or words to that effect).

not at all							very often
0	1	2	3	4	5	6	7

My doctors have become irritated with me because I have improved little with treatment.

not at all							very often
0	1	2	3	4	5	6	7

To score this exercise, add up the numbers you circled, then divide by 7. This is your physician criticism of pain score. This number should be between 0 and 7. Put your score on the Pain Scorecard.

Interpreting Your Score

Level three: 1.6 or more.   Look closely at the items on this scale and see if one or two stand out against the rest. My experience has been that physicians do find organic reasons for their patients' pain problems but have exhausted most if not all of their resources to help. Often, the treatments they have offered have not been seen as helpful by their patients. This is when they make a referral to behavioral medicine and psychology services.

However, your physician may believe that organic factors have been ruled out as the cause of the pain and may refer you for psychosocial assessment and treatment, which can unfortunately imply that the pain is all in your head. If this happens, you may turn to other physicians in the hope of finding physical and biological explanations and treatments of the pain. Under such circumstances, you may feel pressure to convince yourself and others that your pain is real. Psychosocial explanations may be unsatisfactory to you because you perceive them as denying that your suffering is rooted in a real bodily experience deserving of medical attention and sympathy.

This pattern—focusing first on biological explanations and treatments, and turning to psychological factors only after the biological approach fails—fuels the desire of pain sufferers and their families for a biologically based diagnosis and solution. The biomedical emphasis on underlying pathology, combined with individuals' and families' desire to avoid the stigma of a psychological explanation, creates a fixation and focus that is solely medical and physical. However, if you reject the biopsychosocial approach, you are missing a powerful opportunity to change your experience of chronic pain.

Take a look also at your scores on the Lack of Medical Comprehensiveness Scale (exercise 5.3) and the Catastrophic Ideas Scale (exercise 8.1). A high score on all three of these scales suggests you need to have a meeting with your physician to discuss your treatment plan.

Level two: 0.4 to 1.5.   Your experience with your physicians is similar to most other people with chronic pain. That this average range is very low reflects the fact that physician criticism of pain does not occur at a very high rate. This is good.

Level one: 0.3 or less.   You have had minimal to no negative experiences with your physicians. This is obviously good. Take a look at your score on the Lack of Medical Comprehensiveness Scale (exercise 5.3) to see if there are any medical concerns you have that should be discussed with your physician.

WHO GETS GOOD PAIN MANAGEMENT?

Regardless of the intentions of physicians, studies have shown that physicians tend to take more seriously those people in acute pain and those with cancer when compared to those with chronic nonmalignant pain. A Michigan study of 368 physicians looked at how patient characteristics influenced physician behaviors (Green et al. 2001). The study found that physicians were more likely to provide optimal treatment for men with acute postoperative or cancer pain. Physicians reported lesser goals for relief of chronic pain when compared to acute and cancer pain.

My own research has suggested that young, white females are the group most likely to feel invalidated by their physicians; they tend to have the highest scores on the Physician Criticism of Pain Scale.

It is important to recognize that physicians respond differently based on personal characteristics. There are many possible reasons for this, but none change the results. It may not be right, but it happens.

What can you do about it? You can't change your gender, race, or age, but you do have some control over how your doctor perceives you—and thus whether you get effective pain care. Many of the potential problems you can encounter arise from the underlying theme of others doubting your trustworthiness or credibility. It's important that you communicate openly with your doctor. Do your best to present yourself as calm and reasonable, especially when you're describing your pain. Share the exercises and graphs in this book with your doctor to show your commitment to participating in your own rehabilitation. Express your commitment to use medication responsibly.

HELPING YOUR PHYSICIANS HELP YOU

Be prepared for your next doctor's appointment by bringing key information, including:

- Completed copies of exercise 4.2, Rate Your Pain over the Past Week, for the week following any medical procedures you've had since the last visit

- Notes about any changes after you started new medications (positive benefits on pain intensity ratings or negative side effects)

- Completed copies of exercise 4.6, Pain Flare-Up Record, as evidence of pain triggers

- Any other graphs or charts you feel are important

- A copy of the medication contract from chapter 7, if long-term medications are being considered.

Communicating assertively with your physician—asking for what you believe you need —will help you achieve more effective pain management. Finally, offer feedback on your progress and acknowledge anything good your doctor does for you. Physicians are human too, and can benefit from positive reinforcement.

TO SUM UP

Physicians play a very important part in your pain experience, but that part is not always positive. You must take an active role in your treatment, just as you do in every other aspect of your life. You are part of the team that is treating your chronic pain.

Part 3 of this book offers some conclusions based on all the work you have done in parts 1 and 2. Part 4 wraps it all up in a neat bundle that describes your personal pain profile.

PART 3

CONCLUSION

In *Future Shock* (1984), Alvin Toffler wrote about the importance of being adaptable and flexible in an ever-changing world. Managing chronic pain is a true test of this ability. By working through this book, you have learned skills to help you be adaptable and apply what you have learned flexibly. That adaptability and flexibility can be carried over to all aspects of your life.

This section is all about maintaining the progress you have achieved and preparing for obstacles in the future. By following the recommendations and techniques in this book, you can reduce your risk for experiencing further pain problems. Similarly, preparing yourself for high-risk situations and stressful times can decrease the frequency, intensity, and duration of your flare-ups.

PERSISTENCE

Like most people with chronic pain, you are probably going to have flare-ups, setbacks, and delays in your self-management program. This is to be expected. Acquiring self-management skills takes time, and mistakes and lapses are common, particularly in the early stages of pain management. Consider such setbacks opportunities for new learning rather than indications of personal failure or lack of motivation.

Toddlers do not learn to walk the first time they try it. They start by crawling and frequently fall to the ground in their early attempts to walk. This doesn't mean they've done anything wrong or that they should feel at all discouraged. It just means they need to keep trying. Persistence pays off.

The most common triggers for pain flare-ups and pain setbacks, and the issues most people need to keep working at, are poor activity pacing, poor body mechanics, unproductive ideas and thoughts regarding pain, and negative emotional states. None of these will change overnight. Knowledge is only the first step. Once you know better, you do better, and you do it again and again and again until the new approaches and thoughts become habit and then second nature. The key is to make a decision every time to do something different.

ANTICIPATING SETBACKS

Now that you've learned some skills, reevaluated your thoughts, and committed to a self-management program, it is time to think about setbacks. What are they? How can you avoid them? If you can't avoid them, how can you handle them?

In terms of chronic pain, a setback is anything that damages your quality of life and interferes with your function and ability to engage in activities of daily living. Setbacks can include drop-offs in activity levels, depression, heightened anxiety, long-term sleep problems, and overreliance on medications.

There are four primary factors that influence setbacks. Each contributes in a different way to exacerbating pain. You might encounter one or more of these problems:

■   You don't practice or use the coping strategies you've learned.

■   You're holding unproductive ideas or beliefs about your condition.

■   Your family isn't supportive.

■   The treatment you're trying just isn't a good match for you.

MEASURING YOUR PROGRESS

When you read chapter 4, you filled out the Discovery Journal (exercise 4.3) for a week, tracking how you felt on a day-to-day basis, and you used the Pain Flare-Up Record (exercise 4.6) to pinpoint the triggers of your flare-ups. Now it's time to take a look at how you have done so far. Fill out these forms again for a week. Then use them to complete the Measuring Your Progress worksheet.

MEASURING YOUR PROGRESS

Compare your Discovery Journal and Pain Flare-Up Records from the beginning with your current week. You have been tracking your pain intensity and the frequency, duration, and number of flare-ups. Have there been any changes?

Look at the Coping Strategies Used section of your Discovery Journal. What coping strategies were you previously using?

What strategies are you using now?

Examine your energy level ratings. How have they changed?

Looking at your original Pain Flare-Up Records, can you identify any particular activities that were recurring triggers?

If so, look through the activity interference and avoidance scales in chapter 10 and find the scale that includes that activity. What was your interference score the first time you filled out that scale?

Fill out that same scale again. What is your interference score now?

Ideally, you have begun to reduce both the frequency of your flare-ups and the intensity and duration of the flare-ups you do have. Perhaps you have learned to manage things that trigger flare-ups. At the same time, you should notice that you are better rested and have higher energy levels.

By occasionally monitoring your progress, you can keep any future pain flare-ups in perspective. Flare-ups don't mean that you have lost all of your self-management skills. The last thing you need is to undermine your own progress by being too hard on yourself.

ACCOMPLISHMENTS

By now you have accomplished a lot by working through this book. Whether your achievements match up with your goals only you can say, but take a moment to realize what you have accomplished.

The three major areas of change are educating yourself, identifying high-risk situations for pain flare-ups, and learning new coping skills. Your goals likely fell into all three categories.

Educating Yourself

Information is power, and that power is now yours. Throughout these pages, you have learned about the following:

- The difference between acute and chronic pain, and how each is treated

- Pain flare-ups and those factors contributing to your pain experience

- Activity pacing as a pain management skill

- Relaxation training

- Managing your mood

- Challenging unproductive ideas about pain

Information alone does not lead to change; you must take action. I hope this book has encouraged you to take the lead in making some changes in your life and in the way you cope with pain.

Identifying High-Risk Situations

Identifying high-risk situations for pain flare-ups involves noticing early indicators of controllable pain triggers. You should be able to identify your high-risk situations. By now you know the specific set of conditions that have the greatest association with pain for you. These conditions may include:

- High-risk states: certain times of day, boredom, idle time

- Pain behaviors: bracing yourself, clenching your teeth, limping, poor posture, feeling stiff and tense

- Problematic ideas and thoughts about pain: catastrophic thinking, fear of reinjury, future despair

- Mood changes: depression, loneliness, anger, boredom

Learning New Strategies

Throughout this book, you have developed new tools, behaviors, and strategies that will help you make progress in managing your pain.

Effective coping skills.   You have practiced breathing exercises, activity pacing, challenging unproductive ideas and thoughts about pain, and other coping techniques. You are more familiar with how to set realistic specific, positive, and achievable goals.

New lifestyle behaviors that support pain management.   Making positive changes in your leisure, recreational, and employment activities can help reduce pain flare-ups.

Increased self-efficacy.   In this context, *self-efficacy* is the belief that you can improve your pain experience. Each time you enter a high-risk situation for pain, you choose your response based on your appraisal of your ability to cope with the situation. If you view yourself as competent, you will make choices that reduce the likelihood of increased pain. If you don't consider yourself competent, you are at increased risk for pain flare-ups. You have gradually learned to enter high-risk situations and use new responses. Now it's time to trust what you've learned.

Reframing.   Seeing a flare-up as an opportunity to learn and practice new skills (instead of as a catastrophe) reduces the shame and sense of failure often experienced by people in pain.

Daily monitoring.   Monitoring your progress keeps you engaged and helps you analyze your progress. You've learned to use worksheets that give you a clear, tangible measure of the effectiveness of your pain self-management program.

TROUBLESHOOTING

If you decide you have not met some of your pain management goals, then try to pinpoint likely reasons. Here are some possibilities:

- Your initial assessment of your readiness and intention to change (which we discussed in chapter 3) was not accurate, in which case you may need to take the time to look deep into yourself and genuinely commit to making changes.

- You need to discuss your pain management approach with your physician or health care provider to determine a more appropriate course of action.

■ Your pain management strategies require a longer time to take effect. This doesn't necessarily mean your approach will be unsuccessful; it may simply mean that you need to continue with the program.

■ Your approach is appropriate, but the amount of time you have invested has not been sufficient. Try putting more time into the program.

MAINTAINING YOUR GAINS AND AVOIDING SETBACKS

If you have reached your goals in your pain self-management program, you'll need to put some energy into maintaining your success. Keep in mind the following:

■ Pain is part of everyday life and is experienced by everyone. Acute pain is a useful signal that something is wrong. Chronic pain is not. While acute pain is a warning to stop what you are doing, chronic pain may mean you have to keep moving.

■ Rather than allowing yourself to become overwhelmed with pain, use the monitoring forms in this book to objectively evaluate the triggers that launched the flare-up, understand the sequencing of events, and modify your behavior.

■ Try not to allow yourself to fall into the pattern that chronic pain typically teaches: rest, lie down, avoid activities, be afraid, isolate yourself. Don't let chronic pain limit your life.

You can prevent or minimize future pain setbacks by preparing for them. Identify situations that put you at increased risk for a flare-up. Have a plan in place. Be ready to use the tools you've learned, such as belly breathing, coping statements written on a card in your wallet or purse, and an activity pacing timer. Include family members in your plan. Join a support group.

Here are some do's and don'ts for maintaining your gains.

Do remember that the changes you are attempting to make are part of a bigger picture of overall health and well-being and that it takes small but steady steps to reach this goal.

Do realize that even after trying the suggestions in this book, you may sometimes have trouble managing your pain. Contacting health care professionals to assist you in managing your pain is not a sign of failure.

Do revisit the scales in this book to measure changes (positive or negative) from your original score. Use this as a progress report card. This will also refresh your memory about the skills you have learned.

Do realize that you may not need to continue your initial pain management regimen once you reach a certain healthy level of functioning. For example, family and friends may no longer need to be reminded to avoid behaviors that perpetuate or maintain your pain. Once you achieve a certain level of physical activity, you no longer need to continue increasing this level. Once you're off narcotic medications, you no longer have to go through withdrawals. It may be enough to continue some pain management strategies only as needed.

Do participate in pain management support groups for booster sessions when needed. Go to the chat group off my Web site at www.PainCareWorkbook.com and talk to others who have read *The Chronic Pain Care Workbook*. See what has worked for them.

Do involve family members by having them read sections of this book to understand what you are trying to accomplish with the self-management approach to pain.

Do seek assistance and guidance from a clinician in such areas as setting up an appropriate exercise program or addressing long-standing family or marital conflicts that may be worsened by your chronic pain problem.

Don't conclude that any future pain flare-up is an indication of personal failure or inability to cope. Future flare-ups are opportunities to practice what you have learned and prove to yourself that you do have the power to reduce flare-ups before they get out of control.

Don't fall into the "-izing" trap. Catastrophizing, overgeneralizing, "awfulizing," and personalizing are all traps that can perpetuate the pain experience.

Don't attribute all of life's problems and stress to your pain. Learn to distinguish between your pain and other emotional problems. Determine which problems are directly related to your pain and which are related to other things. This way, you can address pain problems with pain management strategies and tackle other problems (family, marital, or employment issues) with other strategies.

COMING TO TERMS WITH CHRONIC PAIN

Pain management is making strides to assist millions of people suffering from chronic pain. By understanding what influences your pain and learning ways to improve your pain experience, you can live a better life.

I have presented an effective model for understanding chronic pain: the biopsychosocial perspective. Each component of this model offers strategies for enhancing your pain management skills. The exercises in this book have helped you gather the information you need to tailor your treatment to match your individual characteristics and response to pain. One size does not fit all when it comes to pain treatment. People with different characteristics will likely benefit from different treatment (Turk 1990).

You have taken a journey to understand the complex phenomenon of chronic pain. The journey is also one into yourself, into a deeper understanding of your pain and your experience of that pain.

Two primary goals of the pain self-management approach are improved quality of life and enhanced ability to function and engage in life's daily activities. I hope you now feel well equipped with ideas and strategies to accomplish these two primary goals. You can keep enjoyable activities in your life and pursue meaningful pleasures. I hope that as you look toward the future, you feel more empowered and better able to take on whatever chronic pain will present to you. You now have a set of skills to help you cope.

I hope that the people you have read about in the stories in this book will inspire you and help you appreciate the hard work and tenacity it takes to make positive changes in your life with pain. These changes can be made, as proved by those who have walked the path before you.

I hope working through this book has been a validating and affirming experience. God knows people in chronic pain need all of that. I also hope you have been able to see the ways you have already been coping well with your pain (as evidenced by your level one scores on the Pain Scorecard). Remember to pat yourself on the back and affirm the positive.

Now get moving.

PART 4

YOUR PAIN SCORECARD

In this section, you'll record your scores from the scales throughout the book. I'll guide you in interpreting this information to understand your strengths and areas of concern for pain management. Finally, I'll provide treatment suggestions targeted for specific areas of concern.

CREATING YOUR PAIN SCORECARD

For each scale, circle the range that includes your score. The first time you complete the exercise, write your score in the "before" column. When you take a scale again, write your score in the "after" column.

	Level One: Minimal Impact (These are your personal strengths in coping with chronic pain.)	Level Two: Moderate Impact (These are your areas of moderate concern. Suggestions in this book should be very helpful.)	Level Three: Significant Negative Impact (These are your areas of significant concern. Focus your energy here first. Assistance from a clinician is recommended.)	Before Score	After Score
Rate Your Pain over the Past Week (exercise 4.2)	0–10	11–20 *17*	21–30		
Lack of Medical Comprehensive-ness Scale (exercise 5.3)	0–2.3	2.4–4.1	4.2–7.0		
Reduced Productivity Scale (exercise 6.5)	0–2.6	2.7–4.8	4.9–7.0		
Sleep Interference Scale (exercise 6.6)	0–2	3–4	5–9		
Muscular Discomfort Scale (exercise 6.8)	0–3.3	3.4–4.9	5.0–7.0		
Catastrophic Ideas Scale (exercise 8.1)	0–1.9	2.0–3.6	3.7–7.0		
Fear of Reinjury Scale (exercise 8.4)	0–3.1	3.2–5.0	5.1–7.0		
Entitlement/ Frustration Scale (exercise 8.6)	0–4.2	4.3–5.4	5.5–7.0		

Self-Blame Scale (exercise 8.7)	0–1.7	1.8–3.4	3.5–7.0		
Future Despair Scale (exercise 8.8)	0–1.3	1.4–3.4	3.5–7.0		
Social Disbelief Scale (exercise 8.9)	0–0.6	0.7–2.3	2.4–7.0		
Pain Behaviors Scale (exercise 9.1)	0–2.9	3.0–4.2	4.3–7.0		
Interference and Avoidance Scale for Domestic Activities (exercise 10.1)	interference: 0–1.0	interference: 1.1–2.6	interference: 2.7–7.0		
	avoidance: 0–2.6	avoidance: 2.7–4.5	avoidance: 4.6–7.0		
Interference and Avoidance Scale for Physically Demanding Activities (exercise 10.3)	interference: 0–1.8	interference: 1.9–3.4	interference: 3.5–7.0		
	avoidance: 0–3.4	avoidance: 3.5–5.5	avoidance: 5.6–7.0		
Interference and Avoidance Scale for Social Activities (exercise 10.5)	interference: 0–0.6	interference: 0.7–2.3	interference: 2.4–7.0		
	avoidance: 0–2.4	avoidance: 2.5–4.5	avoidance: 4.6–7.0		
Interference and Avoidance Scale for Personal Care Activities (exercise 10.7)	interference: 0–1.1	interference: 1.2–2.5	interference: 2.6–7.0		
	avoidance: 0–2.3	avoidance: 2.4–4.0	avoidance: 4.1–7.0		
Interference and Avoidance Scale for Personal Hygiene Activities (exercise 10.9)	interference: 0–0.1	interference: 0.2–0.8	interference: 0.9–7.0		
	avoidance: 0–0.6	avoidance: 0.7–2.3	avoidance: 2.4–7.0		

Anticipated Emotional Distress Scale (exercise 11.1)	0–1.4	1.5–3.3	3.4–7.0		
Depression Scale (exercise 11.2)	0–1.6	1.7–3.3	3.4–7.0		
Fear of Pain Scale (exercise 11.3)	0–3.3	3.4–5.4	5.5–7.0		
Anxiety Scale (exercise 11.4)	0–1.5	1.6–3.0	3.1–7.0		
Relationship Interference Scale (exercise 12.1)	0–2.0	2.1–4.1	4.2–7.0		
Partner Criticism of Pain Scale (exercise 12.4)	0–0.4	0.5–1.7	1.8–7.0		
Partner Reinforcement of Pain Scale (exercise 12.5)	0–2.5	2.6–4.4	4.5–7.0		
Partner Discouragement of Wellness Scale (exercise 12.6)	0–2.2	2.3–4.3	4.4–7.0		
Partner Reinforcement of Wellness Scale (exercise 12.7)	4.1–7.0	2.4–4.0	0–2.3		
Physician Reinforcement of Wellness Scale (exercise 14.1)	4.0–7.0	2.1–3.9	0–2.0		
Physician Discouragement of Wellness Scale (exercise 14.2)	0–1.3	1.4–2.8	2.9–7.0		
Physician Criticism of Pain Scale (exercise 14.3)	0–0.3	0.4–1.5	1.6–7.0		

UNDERSTANDING YOUR PAIN SCORECARD

People who experience chronic pain do so in markedly different ways. As you've learned, pain can begin in a variety of ways and can be maintained and aggravated by biological, psychological, and social factors. Constellations of physical, emotional, behavioral, and social factors can vary from person to person.

One of the primary goals of *The Chronic Pain Care Workbook* has been to assess your unique pain problem using the biopsychosocial model. By completing the scales throughout the book, you have gathered the information to create your pain profile. Now you're ready to identify your personal strengths and areas of concern. In the final section, I'll help you tailor your treatment to meet the needs you've identified.

Your Pain Management Strengths

Review your Pain Scorecard and find all the areas in which you scored at level one. Write them here:

These are your personal strengths in your pain self-management program. You can draw some conclusions from the particular areas in which you're doing well. For example, if you scored in level one on catastrophic ideas, fear of reinjury, lack of medical comprehensiveness, and partner reinforcement of wellness, we could conclude that you are not using black-and-white thinking, you are not feeling out of control of your life, you are not fearful of hurting yourself, you believe that your medical treatment has been comprehensive, and you have a supportive partner who encourages you in your wellness activities. Remember to accept the positive and pat yourself on the back for your strengths.

Your Areas of Moderate Concern

Below, list all the areas in which you scored at level two.

These are your areas of moderate concern. The self-management approaches you've learned in this book may be quite helpful in addressing these problems. But first, you'll need to focus on the more serious concerns.

Your Most Significant Areas of Concern

List all the scales on which you scored at level three below:

These are the areas where you need to concentrate your time, energy, and effort. Before we discuss treatment approaches, we'll create a different kind of overview of your scores.

ARRANGING YOUR SCORES BY CATEGORY

Let's consider whether a particular category—biological, psychological, or social—stands out as an area of concern for you.

Biological

Check the boxes for any scales on which you scored at level three.

☐   Lack of Medical Comprehensiveness Scale

☐   Rate Your Pain over the Past Week

☐   Muscular Discomfort Scale

☐   Pain Behaviors Scale

☐   Interference Scale for Domestic Activities

☐   Avoidance Scale for Domestic Activities

☐   Interference Scale for Physically Demanding Activities

☐   Avoidance Scale for Physically Demanding Activities

☐   Interference Scale for Social Activities

☐   Avoidance Scale for Social Activities

☐   Interference Scale for Personal Care Activities

☐   Avoidance Scale for Personal Care Activities

☐   Interference Scale for Personal Hygiene Activities

☐   Avoidance Scale for Personal Hygiene Activities

☐   Sleep Interference Scale

Add up the number of boxes you checked above, divide by 15, and write this number as a percentage under "Biological" in the table at the end of this section.

Psychological

Check the boxes for any scales on which you scored at level three.

☐   Depression Scale

☐   Fear of Pain Scale

☐   Anxiety Scale

☐   Catastrophic Ideas Scale

☐   Fear of Reinjury Scale

☐   Entitlement/Frustration Scale

Add up the number of boxes you checked above, divide by 6, and write this number as a percentage under "Psychological."

Social

Check the boxes for any scales on which you scored at level three.

☐   Social Disbelief Scale

☐   Partner Reinforcement of Pain Scale

☐   Partner Criticism of Pain Scale

☐   Partner Discouragement of Wellness Scale

☐   Physician Reinforcement of Wellness Scale

☐   Physician Criticism of Pain Scale

☐   Physician Discouragement of Wellness Scale

Add up the number of boxes you checked above, divide by 7, and write this number as a percentage under "Social."

Percentages of Level Three Scores by Category		
Biological	Psychological	Social

Once you have identified your area of greatest concern—biological, psychological, or social—you can focus your treatment efforts there as a starting point. Then you can move on to the next highest category, then the next. The treatment recommendations at the end of this chapter are divided into these three categories.

WHERE YOU'VE BEEN, WHERE YOU ARE: THE BIG PICTURE

In chapter 2, you completed the pain circle exercise, where you filled in a circle to show how much of your pain experience reflected biological, psychological, and social influences. Now consider the following:

- Has that circle changed its proportions since you've read the book and taken the various surveys?

- Has one area of the biopsychosocial model changed in its importance, or have they stayed the same?

- Have you been surprised by any of your responses to the questions or by the implications of any of your scores?

SELF-MANAGEMENT SUGGESTIONS FOR COMMON AREAS OF CONCERN

This table lays out common thoughts, questions, and areas of concern and offers treatment suggestions related to each. Use this information to focus your treatment efforts.

Question, Thought, or Area of Concern	Action Plan
Physical/Biological	
What is causing my pain? *Why do I have pain?* *I don't know my diagnosis.* *I don't know what is causing my pain.*	▪ Have your physician present your diagnosis and the possible causes, preferably in writing. ▪ Get copies of all your medical records. ▪ Explore treatment options with health care staff. ▪ Determine what isn't your diagnosis. This will help you reduce your fears and avoid catastrophizing. ▪ Contact pain support groups. ▪ Know what the medical guidelines are for treating this condition.
I have not been treated comprehensively or completely.	▪ Review your concerns with your current physician. ▪ Write down what you think needs to be done to help you with your pain problem. Be specific. Don't simply say, "I just want my pain to be gone." Discuss with your doctor what treatments (such as physical therapy, occupational therapy, depression management, medications, or surgery) would help with your pain. ▪ Seek a second opinion, perhaps from a physician in a different specialty than that of your treating physician. ▪ Ask yourself how many doctors you have seen and how many is enough. ▪ Consider the idea that your best bet is to manage pain and increase your function and quality of life, rather than expecting a cure.
What do I do when I have a bad pain flare-up?	▪ Work out ahead of time with your physician what you should do if your pain gets out of control. ▪ Review your positive coping statements. ▪ Remember to employ coping strategies early on, as the flare-up starts, not during the peak of the pain.

My pain medications are not working. *It takes too long for my medications to work.* *The level of pain relief provided by my medications is not satisfactory.* *The relief from my pain medications does not last long enough.* *I am worried about taking my current pain medication for a long time.* *My medications are not good for my physical health.* *My medications do not allow me to perform my daily activities the way I want to.* *My medications are not helping my mood, and my quality of life is not acceptable.* *My medications are limiting my ability to concentrate.* *My relationships with others have not improved even though I'm taking my medications.*	▨ Consult your physician and pharmacist for information about your medications. ▨ Ask your physician about other medication options. Find out whether you are a candidate for long-term opioid analgesic treatment, time-released medications for pain, or medications from different classes. ▨ Are you taking the medications as directed? Many people do not, and then conclude the medications aren't working. Make sure you give your medications a chance to work. For example, some antidepressants can take up to two or three months to give their full benefit. ▨ Consider taking the Sample Medication Contract from chapter 7 to your physician.
I think I need diagnostic testing. *I need more testing.*	▨ What diagnostic testing have you had? ▨ When was your last test? If it was just a month ago, perhaps not much has changed that would show up on tests. If it has been years, ask your physician about diagnostic testing.
I need more treatment.	▨ List what you think should be done and hasn't, and bring this list to your doctor. ▨ Keep good records of all treatments and reports. ▨ Ask yourself whether you have experienced any improvement from a specific treatment. If not, it may be hard to argue for more treatment.

I have trouble falling asleep. *I wake up frequently throughout the night.* *I sleep less overall.* *I don't wake up rested and refreshed.*	▪ Read the Sleep, Energy, and Chronic Pain section of chapter 6. ▪ Learn relaxation skills, guided imagery, and visualization techniques to quiet yourself before sleep. ▪ Practice getting out of bed if you don't fall asleep after ten to fifteen minutes in bed.
fatigue, low energy *activity avoidance*	▪ Ask yourself whether you are an "overdoer" or an "underdoer." ▪ Pace yourself with appropriate activity levels.
pain or difficulty with sexual activity	▪ Check with a physical therapist on body positions and pain recommendations. ▪ Examine your use and timing of medications and the impact on your desire and capacity to function. ▪ Practice communication skills.
using caffeine (coffee, tea, soda)	▪ Try cutting back. Caffeine may increase agitation and aggravate anxiety, ultimately increasing pain perception.
using nicotine	▪ Quit smoking. Seek help if you need it.
using alcohol	▪ Reduce or eliminate your use of alcohol. It can disturb your sleep patterns. Alcohol use is essentially a passive coping strategy for pain management. Try using active, healthy strategies instead.
Psychological/Emotional	
not ready to think about change	▪ Hang on to this book for future reference.
catastrophic ideas	▪ Seek cognitive behavioral therapy that emphasizes modifying unproductive ideas about pain. ▪ Use the Thought Evaluation Form from chapter 8.

fears of reinjury	■ Try graduated increases in physical activities. ■ Try the relaxation techniques from chapter 6. ■ Use the Thought Evaluation Form to challenge any unrealistic ideas you have about reinjuring yourself.
expecting a cure	■ Try cognitive behavioral therapy. ■ Hang on to this book for future reference.
self-blame	■ Seek mood and depression management.
entitlement/frustration	■ Seek assertiveness training. ■ Seek anger management.
depression	■ Try cognitive behavioral therapy. ■ Increase pleasant activities. ■ Consult with your physician.
anxiety	■ Try relaxation training. ■ Use progressive muscle relaxation. ■ Use guided imagery.
anger	■ Seek assertiveness training and anger management.
productivity interference	■ Use activity pacing to reach acceptable levels of activity. ■ Begin a graduated exercise plan. ■ Explore perfectionistic traits and rigidity. ■ Learn and practice relaxation skills.
fear of pain *fear of physical harm*	■ Ask yourself how you want to be different and compare that with your goals. Do they match? ■ Seek anxiety treatment. ■ Work on stress management. ■ Start a graduated movement program. ■ Use activity pacing.
Social	
conflict with spouse, family, or loved ones	■ Explore coping strategies in communication skills, assertiveness, positive parenting.

No one believes my pain is as bad as it is.	■ Talk with your loved ones about your feeling that your pain experience is being invalidated. ■ Ask your family what they think and feel about your pain. ■ Recognize that pain is invisible and cannot be seen by others. ■ Consider the idea that you don't have to prove anything to anyone.
I don't like going to work anymore. I miss going to work.	■ Enjoying the tasks of your job is a strong predictor of return to work. If you don't enjoy your job (or the job you had most recently), consider this an opportunity to explore a new line of work. ■ Work on communication skills and assertiveness. ■ How well you like and get along with coworkers often determines job satisfaction. Cultivate friendships in your workplace.
I want my sex life back.	■ Work on more effective communication skills. ■ Differentiate between sensuality and sexuality.

If any of these treatment suggestions sound overwhelming or impossible, remember that you can seek professional assistance from a doctor or therapist. You don't ever have to go it alone. Consider bringing this Pain Scorecard with you to share what work you have been doing in your pain self-management program.

Resources

Improving your chronic pain experience is your responsibility, but that doesn't mean you need to go it alone. The following are just some of the resources out there to help you.

SUPPORT GROUPS FOR PEOPLE WITH CHRONIC PAIN

Support groups can provide help, advice, and, of course, support that you cannot find anywhere else. The people participating in these groups share many of the same symptoms and feelings you have. But not all support groups are the same. Some are educational, and some are more social. The major benefits of joining a support group include a sense that you are not alone; others also suffer from chronic pain. This can be very therapeutic in itself. You can feel understood by others and share a sense of camaraderie. Ideally, once you experience being accepted just as you are, you begin to feel more accepting toward yourself. You can also share your unique experiences with the group and perhaps learn from what others have gone through.

Support groups can be counterproductive if they become too negative and angry. Focusing on the negative can bring you down and defeat the primary purpose of the group, which is to support the members.

The American Chronic Pain Association offers listings of local support groups. The ACPA can also provide information about starting a support group if there isn't one in your community.

American Chronic Pain Association
(800) 533-3231
www.theacpa.org

INFORMATION ABOUT CHRONIC PAIN AND ITS TREATMENT

American Academy of Family Physicians
www.familydoctor.org

American Pain Foundation
www.painfoundation.org

Mayday Pain Project
www.painandhealth.org

Mayo Clinic
www.mayoclinic.org

National Guideline Clearinghouse
www.guideline.gov

National Institutes of Health
www.nih.gov

National Network of Libraries of Medicine
http://nnlm.gov

National Pain Foundation
www.painconnection.org

Thomson Healthcare PDR
www.pdrhealth.com

PAIN CONDITIONS

American Council for Headache Education
www.achenet.org

Arthritis Foundation
www.arthritis.org

National Fibromyalgia Association
www.fmaware.org

National Institute of Arthritis and Musculoskeletal and Skin Diseases
www.niams.nih.gov

National Institute of Dental and Craniofacial Research (NIDCR)
www.nidcr.nih.gov

National Institute of Neurological Disorders and Stroke (NINDS): includes information about peripheral neuropathy, reflex sympathetic dystrophy syndrome, shingles, and trigeminal neuralgia
www.ninds.nih.gov

NINDS Central Pain Syndrome Information Page
www.ninds.nih.gov/health_and_medical/disorders/centpain_doc.htm

FINDING PAIN CARE PROVIDERS

American Academy of Pain Management
www.aapainmanage.org

American Academy of Pain Medicine
www.painmed.org

American Physical Therapy Association
www.apta.org

American Psychological Association
www.apa.org

Association for Applied Psychophysiology and Biofeedback
www.aapb.org

Commission on Accreditation of Rehabilitation Facilities
www.carf.org

MEDICATIONS

MedlinePlus
www.nlm.nih.gov/medlineplus/druginfo

HEALTHIER LIVING

Exercise

Exercise: A Guide from the National Institute on Aging
http://weboflife.ksc.nasa.gov/exerciseandaging/cover.html

Sleep

Currie, Shawn, and Keith Wilson. 2003. *60 Second Sleep-Ease: Quick Tips for Getting a Good Night's Rest*. Far Hills, NJ: New Horizon Press.

National Institutes of Health: Sleep Disorders Information
www.nhlbi.nih.gov/health/public/sleep

Challenging Unproductive Thinking

Seligman, Martin. 2002. *Authentic Happiness*. New York: Free Press.

Depression

Burns, David. 1999. *Feeling Good: The New Mood Therapy*. New York: Avon Books.

Humor

Cousins, Norman. 1979. *Anatomy of an Illness as Perceived by the Patient*. New York: W. W. Norton & Company.

Sex

Hebert, Lauren. 1997. *Sex and Back Pain: Advice on Restoring Comfortable Sex Lost to Back Pain*. Bangor, ME: IMPACC.

Quitting Smoking

Antonuccio, David. 1992. *Butt Out*. Saratoga, CA: R & E Publishing.

References

Alberti, R. 2001. *Your Perfect Right*. San Luis Obispo, CA: Impact Publisher.

American Chronic Pain Association. 2002. Myths, misunderstanding about pain common among Americans. *Partners for Understanding Pain*, September 17, 1–8.

Beck, J. 1996. *Worksheet Packet*. Bala Cynwyd, PA: Beck Institute for Cognitive Therapy and Research.

Berk, R. A. 2001. The active ingredients in humor: Psychophysiological benefits and risks for older adults. *Educational Gerontology* 27:323–39.

Bortz, W. M. 1984. The disuse syndrome. *Western Journal of Medicine* 141:691–94.

Buer, N., and S. J. Linton. 2002. Fear-avoidance beliefs and catastrophizing: Occurrence and risk factor in back pain and ADL in the general population. *Pain* 99:485–91.

Corcoran, P. J. 1991. Use it or lose it: The hazards of bed rest and inactivity. *Western Journal of Medicine* 154:536–38.

Currie, S. R., K. G. Wilson, A. J. Pontefract, and L. deLaplante. 2000. Cognitive behavioral treatment of insomnia secondary to chronic pain. *Journal of Consulting and Clinical Psychology* 68:407–16.

Elliott, A. M., B. H. Smith, K. Penny, W. L. Smith, and W. A. Chambers. 1999. The epidemiology of chronic pain in the community. *Lancet* 354:1248–52.

Ellis, A., and R. A. Harper. 1975. A *Guide to Rational Living*. Chatsworth, CA: Wilshire Book Company.

Engle, G. L. 1977. The need for a new medical model: A challenge for biomedicine. *Science* 196:129–36.

Fishban, D. A., R. Cutler, H. L. Rosomoff, and R. S. Rosomoff. 1997. Chronic pain–associated depression: Antecedent or consequence of chronic pain? *Clinical Journal of Pain* 13:116–37.

Fishman, S. 2000. *The War on Pain*. New York: HarperCollins.

Flor, H., C. Breitenstein, N. Birbaumer, and M. Furst. 1995. A psychophysiological analysis of spouse solicitousness toward pain behaviors, spouse interaction, and pain perception. *Behavior Therapy* 26:255–72.

Fordyce, W. 1976. *Behavioral Methods for Chronic Pain and Illness.* St. Louis: C. V. Mosby.

Green, C. R., J. R. Wheeler, B. Marchant, F. LaPorte, and E. Guerrero. 2001. Analysis of the physician variable in pain management. *Pain Medicine* 2:317–27.

Hayden, J. A., M. W. van Tulder, A. Malmivaara, and B. W. Koes. 2005. Exercise therapy for treatment of nonspecific low back pain. *The Cochrane Database of Systematic Reviews.* DOI: 10.1002/14651858.CD000335.pub2.

Jasmin, L., D. Tien, G. Janni, and P. T. Ohara. 2003. Is noradrenaline a significant factor in the analgesic effect of antidepressants? *Pain* 106:3–8.

Jensen, M., and D. Patterson. 2006. Hypnotic treatment of chronic pain. *Journal of Behavioral Medicine* 29:95–124.

Kerns, R., R. Rosenberg, and M. Jacob. 1994. Anger expression and chronic pain. *Journal of Behavioral Medicine* 17:57–67.

Kerns, R., R. Rosenberg, R. N. Jamison, M. A. Caudill, and J. A. Haythornthwaite. 1997. Readiness to adopt a self-management approach to chronic pain: The Pain Stages of Change Questionnaire (PSOCQ). *Pain* 72:227–34.

Kessler, R. C., P. Burglund, O. Demler, R. Jin, D. Koretz, K. R. Merikangas, A. J. Rush, E. E. Walters, and P. S. Wang. 2003. The epidemiology of major depressive disorder: Results from the National Comorbidity Survey Replication (NCS-R). *Journal of the American Medical Association* 289:3095–3105.

McCracken, L. M. 1997. "Attention" to pain in persons with chronic pain: A behavioral approach. *Behavior Therapy* 28:271–84.

Melzack, R., and P. D. Wall. 1988. *The Challenge of Pain.* London: Penguin Books.

Morin, C. 1993. *Insomnia: Psychological Assessment and Management.* New York: Guilford Press.

Nevo, O., G. Keinan, and M. Teshimovsky-Arditi. 1993. Humor and pain tolerance. *Humor: International Journal of Humor Research* 6:71–88.

Nicassio, P. M., and K. A. Wallston. 1992. Longitudinal relationships among pain, sleep problems, and depression in rheumatoid arthritis. *Journal of Abnormal Psychology* 101:514–20.

Philips, H. C. 1988. Avoidance behaviour and its role in sustaining chronic pain. *Behaviour Research and Therapy* 25:273–79.

Prochaska, J. O. 1984. *Systems of Psychotherapy: A Transtheoretical Analysis.* Homewood, IL: Dorsey Press.

Prochaska, J. O., and C. C. DiClemente. 1983. Stages and processes of self-change of smoking: Toward an integrative model of change. *Journal of Consulting and Clinical Psychology* 51:390–95.

Romano, J. M., J. A. Turner, L. S. Friedman, R. A. Bulcroft, M. P. Jensen, H. Hops, and S. F. Wright. 1995. Chronic pain patient–spouse behavioral interactions predict pain disability. *Pain* 63:353–60.

Smith, T., and A. Christensen. 1992. Hostility, health, and social contexts. In *Hostility, Coping, and Health,* edited by H. Friedman. Washington, DC: American Psychological Association.

Smith, M. T., R. R. Edwards, R. C. Robinson, and R. H. Dworkin. 2004. Suicidal ideation, plans, and attempts in chronic pain patients: Factors associated with increased risk. *Pain* 111:201–8.

Spielman, A. J., P. Saskin, and M. J. Thorpy. 1987. Treatment of chronic insomnia by restriction of time in bed. *Sleep* 10:45–56.

Suinn, R. M. 2001. The terrible twos—anger and anxiety: Hazardous to your health. *American Psychologist* 56:27–36.

Sullivan, M. J. L., K. Reesor, S. F. Mikail, and R. Fisher. 1992. The treatment of depression in chronic low back pain: Review and recommendations. *Pain* 50:5–13.

Toffler, A. 1984. *Future Shock.* New York: Bantam Doubleday, Dell Publishing Group.

Turk, D. C. 1990. Customizing treatment for chronic pain patients: Who, what, and why. *Clinical Journal of Pain* 6:255–70.

Vlaeyen, J. W. S., and S. J. Linton. 2000. Fear-avoidance and its consequences in chronic musculoskeletal pain: A state of the art. *Pain* 85:317–32.

Waddell, G., M. Newton, I. Henderson, D. Somerville, and C. Main. 1993. A Fear-Avoidance Beliefs Questionnaire (FABQ) and the role of fear-avoidance beliefs in chronic low back pain and disability. *Pain* 52:157–68.

Webster, L. R., and R. M. Webster. 2005. Predicting aberrant behaviors in opioid-treated patients: Preliminary validation of the Opioid Risk Tool. *Pain Medicine* 6:432.

Williams, D. A., M. E. Robinson, and M. E. Geisser. 1994. Pain beliefs: Assessment and utility. *Pain* 59:71–78.

Michael J. Lewandowski, Ph.D., is a licensed psychologist and is president of Pain Assessment Resources. He has extensive training and experience in the application of psychological principles to problems in medicine. Since completing his Ph.D. in 1990, he has worked exclusively with individuals suffering from chronic medical conditions starting during his internship at the Veterans Administration Hospital in Reno, NV. Of the two accredited pain programs in northern Nevada, he helped develop and direct both. He was deemed an expert in chronic pain by the Nevada District Court and has testified in cases in which the validity of chronic pain was questioned. In addition to his clinical, administrative, and legal experience working with chronic pain sufferers, Lewandowski has conducted, presented, and published original scientific research in the area of chronic pain and has presented at national pain conferences throughout the world.

He was principal developer of the Behavioral Assessment of Pain Medical Stability Quick Screen (BAP-MSQS) and codeveloper of the Behavioral Assessment of Pain questionnaire (BAP), which are both utilized in pain management programs around the world. He was co-owner of Integrated Healthcare Resources, an interdisciplinary healthcare organization that provides comprehensive pain management, work hardening, and functional restoration programs for injured workers and persons with chronic pain conditions.

Lewandowski is the secretary/treasurer of the Board of Psychological Examiners for the State of Nevada; a diplomate in the American Academy of Pain Management;; a member of the American Pain Society; and a member of the American Psychological Association. He was licensed as an alcohol and drug abuse counselor by the state of Nevada and is a marriage and family therapist along with being certified as a rehabilitation counselor and biofeedback therapist.

more pain care titles from new**harbinger**publications
real tools for real change since 1973

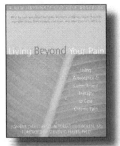

LIVING BEYOND YOUR PAIN
Using Acceptance & Commitment
Therapy to Ease Chronic Pain

a radical new approach to living
well with pain

$19.95 • Item Code: 4097

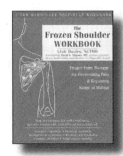

THE FROZEN SHOULDER WORKBOOK
Trigger Point Therapy for Overcoming
Pain & Regaining Range of Motion

powerful techniques for coping with
a common, painful condition

$18.95 • Item Code: 447X

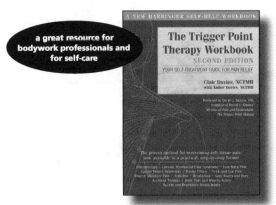

a great resource for
bodywork professionals and
for self-care

THE TRIGGER POINT THERAPY WORKBOOK, SECOND EDITION
Your Self-Treatment Guide for Pain Relief

a powerful collection of gentle massage techniques that target painful
trigger points that occur in the body's soft tissues—highly effective
self-care for chronic pain

$19.95 • Item Code: 3759

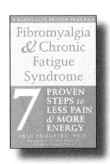

FIBROMYALGIA & CHRONIC FATIGUE
SYNDROME
Seven Proven Steps to Less Pain
& More Energy

a new lifestyle-oriented approach
to living well with FMS and CFS

$14.95 • Item Code: 4593

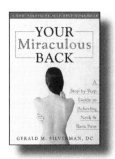

YOUR MIRACULOUS BACK
A Step-by-Step Guide to Relieving
Neck & Back Pain

a safe and sane approach to dealing
with chronic back and neck pain

$18.95 • Item Code: 4526

available from new**harbinger**publications
and fine booksellers everywhere

To order, call toll free **1-800-748-6273**
or visit our online bookstore at **www.newharbinger.com**

(V, MC, AMEX • prices subject to change without notice)